Restful Sleepscape

Unlocking the Secrets of Restful Slumber and Overcoming Insomnia

D. R. Darcy

Table of Contents

Introduction: Embracing the Path to Restful Sleep

Sleep is that golden chain that ties health and our bodies together. – Thomas Decker

Did you know that in 2022, a staggering 21.8% of the US population struggled to find a good night's sleep each and every night? That is over one-fifth of the entire country battling with sleep challenges that disrupt their lives and leave them feeling groggy and exhausted day after day. Let us look at what a dramatic effect this has on the population.

The Problem

As I pondered this astonishing statistic, I could not help but imagine the collective amount of sleep lost by the American population over a year. So, I decided to do some calculations to put it all into perspective.

In a one-year cycle, there are approximately 365 nights. If 21.8% of the US population, which stands at around 332 million people, experiences sleep difficulties every night, we can start to grasp the magnitude of the problem. Multiplying these figures, we find that approximately 72.4 million individuals struggled to sleep each night.

Now, let us consider the amount of sleep lost. The National Sleep Foundation advises adults to have seven to nine hours of sleep nightly, on average. For the sake of this calculation, let us take an average of eight hours of sleep per night. With 72.4 million people losing sleep each night, that amounts to a mind-boggling 579.2 million hours of lost sleep nightly! (Helsestart, n.d.).

Pause for a moment, my fellow insomniac, and let that sink in.

That is over half a billion hours of potential rest and rejuvenation slipping away from the grasp of millions of Americans, night after night. It is an incredible loss, both on an individual level and for society as a whole.

Right, so what is the solution, you ask?

The Solution

In a world that never seems to slow down, where the demands of everyday life push us to our limits, finding a moment of proper rest has become a rare and precious treasure. We live in a society that thrives on hustle and productivity, celebrating those who burn the midnight oil and sacrifice sleep for success.

But at what cost?

In pursuing our dreams and ambitions, we often overlook the importance of rest and its profound impact on our overall well-being. We dismiss it as a luxury or an indulgence, failing to realize that rest is not just a state of inactivity but a vital pillar of a healthy and fulfilling life.

This book is an exploration of that elusive and transformative state: restfulness. It delves into the depths of sleep, relaxation, and rejuvenation, uncovering their power over our bodies, minds, and spirits. It is a celebration of the art and science of rest, an ode to the act of slowing down and nourishing ourselves in a world that urges us to keep pushing forward.

Through a tapestry of stories, research, and practical advice, we will seek to understand the profound significance of restful peace in our lives. From the flickering candlelight of sleep rituals to the cutting-edge discoveries of modern sleep science, we will traverse the landscapes of slumber, exploring the mysteries of our subconscious minds and the intricate dance of hormones that orchestrate our sleep-wake cycles.

But this book is not just about theory or dry scientific facts. It is about *you*, dear reader, and your own personal relationship with rest. It recognizes that each of us carries a unique set of challenges, worries, and desires, and it honors the struggles we face when seeking solace in the comforting arms of sleep.

Sleep matters? Yes, yes, it does!

#SleepMatters

Now, why does this matter? Well, the impact of sleep deprivation goes beyond just feeling tired and irritable. It affects our physical and mental well-being, our productivity, our relationships, and even our safety. Sleep deprivation sufferers have been linked to a proliferated risk of chronic medical issues such as diabetes, obesity, cardiovascular disease, and even mental health issues like depression and anxiety.

But fret not, for this sleeping blueprint guide sheds light on the sleep challenges a significant portion of the world's population faces. It will explore the underlying causes of sleep troubles, offer practical tips and strategies to improve sleep quality, and delve into sleep experts' latest research and insights.

So what makes this book unique?

What to Expect

You can look forward to topics such as:

- **How Dreams Contribute to Restorative Rest:** Unveiling the role of dreams in rejuvenating our minds and bodies during sleep.
- **Overview of the Sleep-Wake Cycle:** Understanding the natural rhythm that governs our sleep and wakefulness.
- **Natural Ways to Boost Melatonin Production:** Exploring techniques and lifestyle changes to enhance the production of the sleep hormone melatonin.
- **Exploring the Power of White Noise:** Harnessing the calming effects of white noise to promote relaxation and improve sleep quality.
- **Techniques for Managing and Treating Sleep Disorders:** Practical strategies for coping with and treating common sleep disorders.
- **The Connection Between Stress, Anxiety, and Sleep Quality:** Uncovering the intricate relationship between stress, anxiety, and sleep quality.
- **Strategies for Reducing Technology Usage Before Bed:** Tips for creating a tech-free wind-down routine to improve sleep hygiene.
- **Strategies for Creating a Consistent Bedtime Routine:** Establishing a personalized routine to signal the body and mind for a restful night's sleep.
- **Exploring the Benefits of Napping for Energy and Cognitive Function:** Discovering the positive effects of strategic daytime napping on energy levels and mental performance.
- **Strategies for Creating Age-Appropriate Sleep Environments and Routines**: Tailoring sleep

environments and routines to suit the specific needs of different age groups.

I am ready; let's go!

Enter the Sanctuary of Sleep

Whether you are someone like me who battles with insomnia, wrestling with a restless mind that refuses to surrender to the night, or a sleep-deprived parent, sacrificing their rest for the sake of your little ones, this book is here to offer solace, guidance, and practical tools to help you reclaim your sleep and rediscover the transformative power of true restfulness.

Take a deep breath and let go of the worries that weigh you down. Prepare for self-discovery as we navigate the labyrinth of sleep disorders, uncover the secrets of creating a sleep sanctuary, and explore the myriad ways to nourish our bodies and minds for restful nights and rejuvenated days.

So, if you are one of the millions struggling to get a good night's sleep or simply curious about the fascinating world of sleep, join me on this enlightening journey. Together, we will uncover the secrets to restful nights and wakeful days, empowering ourselves to reclaim the rest we deserve and the vitality we crave.

Welcome to the realm of restful peace. May this book be your guiding light as you embark on a path of healing, self-care, and rediscovery. Insomniac, it is time to reclaim your right to rest and embrace the profound transformation it can bring to your life.

Chapter 1:

The Power of Quality Sleep

Proper sleep has helped me get to where I am today as an athlete, and it is something that I continue to rely on every day. –Tom Brady

Sleep Science Explained

Sleep, a complex brain-driven process, intrigues researchers globally. It incorporates deep sleep and REM stages, restoring brain memory, consolidating, and regulating functions. Understanding sleep science could reveal its significant effect on our health and well-being.

But what exactly is the significance of sleep in our lives? Picture this for a moment.

Emily, a seven-year-old girl from a small town in Wisconsin, often lies awake at night, her mind buzzing with excitement. She is filled with wonder and curiosity, dreaming of magical worlds and adventurous tales. Although her parents gently encourage her to sleep, they cannot help but smile at her boundless imagination, knowing that her sleepless nights are a testament to her creative spirit.

A few years pass, and now Emily, an 18-year-old high school student living in bustling New York City, is no stranger to sleepless nights. With college applications looming and exams to prepare for, her mind is constantly racing. Late into the night, she studies diligently, fueled by caffeine and determination. Despite the fatigue, she pushes through, knowing that a good night's sleep will elude her until her goals are within reach.

As we jump forward, Emily is now a 35-year-old working professional in London, experiencing sleepless nights as she navigates the challenges of her demanding career and family life. She often finds her mind racing with thoughts and worries when juggling deadlines, meetings, and household responsibilities. She lies in bed each night, hoping for a few moments of respite. She understands the importance of sleep for her well-being, yet the pressures of her daily life make it difficult to find the peace and rest she craves.

By now, Emily is a 65-year-old retiree in a quiet coastal town in California, facing constant battles with sleeplessness. As she enters her golden years, she wakes up frequently throughout the night, her mind occupied by memories and reflections. While she cherishes the wisdom and experiences that come with age, she longs for a whole night's sleep, knowing that it will bring her the rejuvenation and mental clarity she desires to embrace each day fully.

Are you like Emily or the 21.8 million people suffering from restlessness? Did you know the science of sleep could change Emily's life and maybe yours too? Let me explain how.

Sleep, a vital physiological process, influences our health, cognition, and emotional stability, serving as an essential pillar in the architecture of life.

Science

Sleep is a scientific wonder where our brains conduct a symphony of restoration and rejuvenation activities. Distinct sleep stages, unveiled by Electroencephalography (EEG), serve specific purposes. Deep slow-wave sleep fosters physical restoration and energy rejuvenation, while REM sleep, the setting of vivid dreams, boosts our memory consolidation, cognitive development, and creative problem-solving. Sleep regulation, a complex affair, aligns with our internal body clock or circadian rhythm and relies on melatonin, the hormone signaling our bodies to rest as night falls. Each sleep stage enhances our well-being, making sleep an essential part of our lives.

Impact

In a world where sleep was undervalued, individuals overlooked its significant role in their well-being. Sleep, the silent restorative force, was central to their physical and mental health. Nightly, it weaved a refreshing entrancement, promoting tissue repair, stimulating growth, and maintaining metabolism. This mystery charm also enhanced memory, learning, and provided an emotional sanctuary. Despite its benefits, they favored artificial stimulants, ignoring the cognitive and emotional deficits that ensued. As they begun to appreciate sleep's value, they recognized it as a partner, not an adversary, in productivity. It clarified the mind, fortified the body, and nourished the spirit. Acknowledging sleep's pivotal role in health and happiness, they embraced its healing power as night fell, transforming their lives.

As we discovered earlier on, sleep really does matter. But the question is how?

Sleep, often overlooked, is crucial because it boosts our health and well-being. Acting like a skillful artisan, sleep invigorates our physical health by enhancing tissue repair and immunity. Similarly, it works as an efficient librarian, refining our cognitive abilities and memory.

As a therapist, it calms emotional storms, reducing anxiety and depression risks. Beyond that, it balances metabolic regulation, supports weight maintenance, and lessens disease risk. Hence, from a scientific perspective, sleep is a foundational pillar of our health, which we should prioritize daily.

Lack of sleep also has devastating effects on our physical and mental health.

Sleep deprivation impairs bodily repair, disrupts metabolic balance, heightens illness risk, complicates memory and learning, and elevates anxiety and depression. Thus, neglecting sleep can significantly damage physical health and mental resilience.

Going further, I also can't highlight enough the deep connection of sleep with productivity, mood, and cognitive function.

Sleep fortifies cognitive performance through memory organization and enhanced learning. It also balances emotions by easing stress and fostering tranquility. Furthermore, sleep fuels productivity, improving concentration and sparking creativity, while its deficit impairs work outcomes. Hence, sleep is a vital pillar supporting cognition, mood, and efficiency.

The Sleep Stages

Every night initiates a remarkable journey through varied sleep stages, a testament to our body and mind's intricate design. This expedition, from mild starts to deep restorative periods and the realm of dreams, shape a harmonious sleep symphony.

The sleep process is comprised of five distinct phases: wake, N1, N2, N3, and REM. The stages from N1 to N3 belong to non-rapid eye movement (non-REM) sleep, each step signifying an increasingly more profound slumber. Non-REM stages account for about 75% of total sleep, with stage N2 being the most prominent.

Let us look at the functions and characteristics of each sleep stage below.

Wake/Alert Stage: Our brains exhibit high-frequency, low-amplitude beta waves as we awaken. When we relax and close our eyes, the alpha waves take over.

N1 - Light Sleep: Representing 5% of sleep time, N1 is a brief stage where alpha waves give way to low-amplitude mixed-frequency activity, signaling sleep onset.

N2 - Deeper Sleep: Accounting for around 45% of sleep, N2 is when our bodies relax further, marked by sleep spindles and K complexes. These unique brain activities contribute to memory consolidation and sleep maintenance.

N3 - Deepest Non-REM Sleep: With delta waves dominating, N3 represents the deepest level of sleep. Our bodies focus on tissue repair, bone and muscle growth, and immune strengthening during this stage. However, waking from this stage may cause sleep inertia, a temporary period of grogginess.

REM Sleep: REM, comprising around 25% of sleep, is where we dream. Despite skeletal muscles being atonic, the brain remains highly active, similar to wakefulness. During REM, dreaming, rapid eye movements, and irregular muscle activity occur, with each cycle extending in length through the night.

A complete sleep cycle, with each stage from N1 to REM playing a distinct restorative role, is foundational for rejuvenation. Achieving multiple 90- to 110-minute cycles nightly is vital for comprehensive healing, emphasizing the importance of complete sleep cycles for health and well-being (Colten et al., 2006).

Understanding Sleep Needs

Grasping sleep needs, which are crucial for optimal health, productivity, and emotional well-being, entails understanding that different age groups require varying amounts of rest. Awareness of these diverse needs, from newborns to adults, is essential.

Age Group	Required Sleep Duration
Newborns (0–3 months)	14–17 hours scattered during day and nighttime
Infants (4–11 months)	12–15 hours, mostly as naps and during nighttime
Toddlers (1–2 years)	11–14 hours, usually with 1–2 naps during the day
Preschoolers (3–5 years)	10–13 hours. Most kids stop napping by this age.
School-Aged Children (6–13 years)	9–11 hours
Teenagers (14–17 years)	8–10 hours
Adults (18+ years)	7–9 hours. Older adults might require daytime naps.

Lifestyle habits, mental health, chronic conditions, age, and genetics influence individual sleep needs. Recognizing these factors can aid in tailoring schedules to meet personal sleep requirements for overall health and well-being (Olson, 2021).

Here's how to optimize your sleep:

- Start by understanding the recommended sleep hours for your age while also considering your lifestyle factors.
- Monitor your fatigue levels, daytime productivity, and any signs of sleep deprivation.
- Adjust your sleep schedule based on these insights to create a sleep-friendly environment.

- Limit napping to 20–30 minutes, avoid bedtime stimulants, and manage stress to ensure restful nights.

Did You Know?

"Dysania" is characterized by extreme difficulty getting up in the morning, exceeding typical tiredness or grogginess. It is not recognized as a distinct medical diagnosis in its own right, but it is commonly associated with specific physical and mental health conditions.

For instance, dysania often presents in individuals dealing with depression. The depletion of certain neurotransmitters like serotonin and dopamine can make it challenging for people with depression to motivate themselves to get out of bed. The overwhelming feelings of hopelessness and a lack of energy can contribute to this condition.

In addition, dysania can also be linked to certain nutritional deficiencies. For example, an iron deficiency can lead to anemia, which often results in feelings of fatigue and lethargy, making it harder for individuals to leave their beds in the morning.

Dysania may also indicate chronic fatigue syndrome (CFS), a long-term condition that causes persistent fatigue affecting everyday life. People with CFS wake up still feeling tired, regardless of how much sleep they have had.

This condition is complex, and self-diagnosing is not recommended. If you have persistent trouble getting up, it is advised that you consult a medical practitioner to get an accurate diagnosis and appropriate treatment (Cleveland Clinic, 2021).

Unveiling the Benefits of Restful Sleep

Restful sleep goes beyond feeling refreshed. It contributes to overall well-being, invigorating our minds and bodies. During sleep, your body repairs heart and blood vessels and balances hormones. It bolsters the immune system and aids in memory consolidation. A good night's sleep improves focus, mood, and productivity. Embracing sleep's benefits helps us genuinely appreciate this crucial aspect of a balanced, healthy lifestyle.

Did you know most of our body's repair and restoration processes happen when we sleep?

Sleep serves as a repair shop for our bodies and minds. When we journey to the land of nod, our bodies get to work. During this restful state, heart and blood vessels repair and regenerate, supporting cardiovascular health –hormone production peaks, including growth hormones, facilitating cellular renewal and muscle growth. Our immune system becomes more active, fortifying our defenses against disease. As for the brain, it is a time for cleaning and memory consolidation. Toxins get cleared out, and new information and skills are organized and stored, enhancing our cognitive abilities. Thus, sleep is not just a break—it is a vital service station that optimizes our body and mind.

Furthermore, sleep also plays a pivotal role in our ability to learn and in memory consolidation.

Learning

Sleep provides a unique environment that bolsters the brain's capacity for learning. When we sleep, the brain creates stronger neural connections, aiding in acquiring new skills and knowledge. Whether it is mastering a new language, musical instrument, or complex equation, sleep empowers the learning process, boosting our ability to comprehend and retain further information.

Memory Consolidation

Memory consolidation is when our brain stabilizes and stores information gathered during the day. During sleep, specifically during the REM and slow-wave stages, our brain sifts through the day's events, strengthening essential memories and discarding trivial information. As a result, sleep plays a vital role in cementing our memories, enhancing our recall, and, ultimately, shaping our experiences and understanding of the world.

Furthermore, it also influences other areas of our body, including hormone regulation, immune function, and metabolism.

Hormone Regulation

Sleep orchestrates a symphony of hormones, influencing our growth, appetite, and stress response. This includes growth hormones, vital for physical development and tissue repair, which surges during sleep. Leptin and ghrelin, as appetite regulators, also maintain balance while resting. Moreover, sleep mitigates stress by regulating cortisol levels, promoting emotional well-being.

Immune Function

Our immune system utilizes sleep as a tool for defense. During sleep, the body produces infection-fighting substances like cytokines. These help combat foreign invaders, including bacteria and viruses, enhancing our ability to resist infections and recover from illness.

Metabolism

Sleep is crucial in energy utilization and weight management. Lack of sleep can disrupt metabolic processes, including insulin regulation, potentially leading to weight gain and other health issues. So, adequate sleep is critical to maintaining metabolic harmony.

Understanding the Intriguing World of Dreams

Every night, we journey on captivating expeditions into the enigmatic world of dreams. This mysterious empire, where reality intertwines with imagination, mirrors our subconscious uniquely. Deep within the theater of dreams, our minds create intricate narratives filled with symbolism and emotion, offering insights into our deepest desires, fears, and experiences. Truly, understanding our dreams can be like decoding an encrypted message from the depths of our psyche.

Let us quickly look at the purpose and nature of dreams below.

Nature

Dreams, those captivating stories our minds weave while we sleep, are a cornucopia of emotions, images, and experiences. They may replay our daily encounters, bring to life long-forgotten memories, or catapult us into surreal scenarios that defy the laws of physics. Dreams are the magnificent tapestry of our inner being, from serene to nightmarish, imprinted with our personal histories and mental state.

Purpose

Beyond mere nocturnal entertainment, dreams serve critical psychological functions. They're a platform for emotional processing, helping us cope with stressors and traumas. Dreams also contribute to problem-solving and creativity, often providing a unique perspective. Additionally, they are instrumental in memory consolidation, replaying important information, and reinforcing learning. In essence, dreams are our subconscious mind's way of processing life, aiding our mental and emotional wellness.

Many have also theorized in the past as to why they think we dream. Some popular theories include the Activation-Synthesis Hypothesis, Cognitive Theory, Freud's Psychoanalytic Theory, Jung's Collective Unconscious Theory, and Threat Simulation theory.

Freud's Psychoanalytic Theory

Sigmund Freud, the father of psychoanalysis, proposed that dreams are the royal road to the unconscious. He believed dreams serve as a safe space where repressed desires and hidden thoughts can manifest without the constraints of reality. In essence, they are wish-fulfillment narratives that allow us to grapple with our deepest fears and unfulfilled desires (Freud Museum London, n.d.).

Activation-Synthesis Hypothesis

Contrasting with the psychoanalytic approach, the Activation-Synthesis hypothesis by J. Allan Hobson and Robert McCarley suggests dreams result from random neural firing in the brain during REM sleep. Our mind then constructs a story to make sense of these seemingly random signals, resulting in dreams (Happy, 2020).

Cognitive Theory

The Cognitive Theory views dreams as a reflection of our mental capabilities, like problem-solving and memory processing. Dreaming aids in consolidating memories and allows us to process information in novel ways, fostering creativity and learning (Wamsley, 2014).

Jung's Collective Unconscious Theory

Swiss psychiatrist Carl Jung posited that dreams bridge the conscious and unconscious minds, tapping into a universal "collective unconscious" filled with archetypes and symbols common to all humanity. In Jung's view, dreams offer vital insights into personal growth and self-discovery (Fritscher, 2020).

Threat Simulation Theory

Finnish psychologist Antti Revonsuo proposed the Threat Simulation Theory, suggesting that dreams prepare us for potential dangers. By simulating scary scenarios, dreams might have equipped our ancestors with survival strategies, improving their ability to react to real-life threats (Valli & Revonsuo, 2009).

These diverse theories present a multifaceted understanding of why we dream. Whether as expressions of our subconscious desires, coping mechanisms, or cognitive exercises, dreams continue to captivate and confound, reflecting the intricate tapestry of the human mind.

There is also an intricate relationship between the sleep cycle and our dreams.

Dreams mainly occur during the REM sleep phase, creating a unique bond between dreams and the sleep cycle. In REM, the brain's activity increases, closely resembling the wakeful state, sparking the vibrant, story-like dreams we often remember.

Although dreams can occur in non-REM stages, they are typically less detailed and more thought-like. Dreams become more prolonged and intense as the night progresses, with the longest and most vivid dreams happening in the final REM period.

Therefore, getting a whole night's sleep, encompassing multiple REM phases, enhances our dream experiences. Understanding this link between dreams and the sleep cycle underlines the importance of quality sleep for exploring the mysterious world of dreams.

How Dreams Contribute to Restorative Rest

Dreams, the fascinating stories spun in our minds, can remarkably rejuvenate rest, enhancing our emotional and cognitive health. Let us look at how we can explore this in more detail.

Let me explain the role of dreams in emotional regulation and memory processing.

Dreams are extraordinary in emotional regulation, providing a safe harbor for processing emotions. They act as natural therapists, enabling us to confront and resolve emotional matters in a low-risk environment. Unresolved emotional issues often surface in dreams, granting us insights and aiding emotional healing.

Transitioning to memory processing, dreams play a pivotal role here too. They form an essential part of the memory consolidation process, helping to strengthen neural connections related to newly formed memories. Moreover, they assist in "pruning" redundant information, ensuring we retain essential learnings. Thus, our brains effectively manage and store memories through dreaming, contributing to overall cognitive wellness.

Did you know that dream recalls are also connected to our sleep quality?

Sleep quality, a critical facet of overall health, entails several dimensions, including sleep duration, efficiency, and depth. It is not only about how long you sleep but also how well. Sound, uninterrupted sleep fosters effective transitions through sleep stages, particularly REM sleep, where vivid dreaming occurs.

Dream recall, the ability to remember dreams, is closely linked to sleep quality. Typically, a more restful sleep encourages higher dream recall as it allows for extended REM periods. Our brains are active in these periods, creating elaborate narratives that become our dreams.

Therefore, robust sleep quality and dream recall are intrinsically intertwined. Maintaining good sleep hygiene, thus optimizing your sleep quality, increases your chances of remembering your dreams. Hence, tracking your dream recall might even provide insights into your sleep quality, underlining the complex and fascinating interplay between sleep, dreams, and health.

I would like to share some tips on recalling and understanding dreams.

Remembering dreams, an intriguing aspect of sleep, requires a few strategic practices. Firstly, you should maintain a consistent sleep schedule, enhancing your sleep quality and, thus, dream vividness. Additionally, wake up naturally without an alarm, as abrupt awakenings often disrupt the flow of dreams, making them harder to remember.

Upon waking, lay still and give yourself a few moments to recollect your dreams. Rushing out of bed or becoming engrossed in morning tasks can cause dream memories to evaporate quickly. Think about keeping a dream journal by your bed to jot down details as soon as you awaken. Over time, this practice can strengthen your dream recall ability.

Understanding dream content is more subjective and often requires introspection. Some find it helpful to interpret dreams in the context of their daily life experiences or emotional state. Others may turn to theories such as Carl Jung's archetypes or Sigmund Freud's psychoanalytic perspective. Nevertheless, remember that dream interpretation is highly personal, and not all dreams have profound meanings.

Finally, stay open and curious. Navigating the dream world can be fascinating and rewarding, providing unexpected insights into your waking life.

How about trying one (or both) of the remedies below to guide you to those peaceful dreams you are seeking?

Sleep Remedy One: Himalayan Salt and Honey Mix

Are you ready to enhance your sleep naturally? Start with a bit of Himalayan salt under your tongue, gradually letting it melt away. Follow up with a spoonful of unprocessed honey in the same manner. The blend of minerals such as magnesium and potassium in the salt, paired with the natural sugars in honey, fosters a calming atmosphere and aids in creating melatonin. This hormone oversees your sleep cycles.

Sleep Remedy Two: Golden Milk Latte

Warm a cup of your choice of milk—dairy or plant-derived—in a small saucepan, blending in a spoonful of turmeric, a half spoonful of cinnamon, a quarter spoon of ginger, and a slight sprinkle of black pepper. After heating, sweeten with a spoonful of honey. Serve in a cozy mug as a presleep drink for a tranquil, rejuvenating slumber.

Did You Know?

The circadian rhythm, the body's internal clock, controls human sleep patterns, which operate on approximately a 24-hour cycle. It has been found that most people experience two natural periods of maximum sleepiness during the 24-hour day: one between 2 a.m. and 4:00 a.m., and another between 1:00 p.m. and 3:00 p.m., also known as the "post-lunch dip."

The cause for these energy lulls lies in our biology. At these times, the body's internal clock signals sleepiness. It has encouraged many generations across the earth to rest at the hottest part of the day and the darkest part of the night to conserve energy.

While the 2:00 a.m. slump is usually unnoticed (as most people are asleep), the 2:00 p.m. slump is all too familiar. It is often accentuated by eating a large lunch, as blood flow is diverted from the brain to the digestive system, leading to a feeling of lethargy.

Understanding these natural energy dips can help manage daily tasks effectively, saving complex tasks for peak alertness times and doing simpler tasks during natural drops. Napping, exercising, or walking in natural light can also help overcome the afternoon slump (Cleveland Clinic, 2021).

Next up, we will unpack the sleep-wake cycle in more detail. Are you ready, insomniac?

Chapter 2:

Decoding the Sleep-Wake Cycle

Get enough sleep every night. An exhausted mind is rarely productive. – Author Unknown

This chapter dives into the rhythmic dance of the sleep-wake cycle. This universal human experience is as vital as the breath we take. From New York to New Delhi, we will decode this intricate ballet of biology, teasing apart the secrets of your nighttime journey. Are you ready to discover what truly happens when you surrender to the whispers of slumber? Let us embark on this enlightening expedition!

Did You Know?

Indeed, studies have indicated an intriguing connection between the lunar cycle and sleep behavior. It is observed that people tend to sleep less and go to bed later in the few days preceding a full moon. This phenomenon is named "lunar rhythmicity."

Although the exact reasons for this behavior remain unclear, the hypothesis revolves around our ancestral past. Before the advent of artificial lighting, moonlight was a significant source of nighttime illumination. The full moon's brightness may have encouraged our ancestors to stay awake and active, an innate habit that could still persist in our genes.

It is also possible that the moon's gravitational pull could have a subtle impact on human physiology, as it does on the tides, affecting sleep patterns. However, this is a less-explored hypothesis, and more research is needed to establish a clear cause-and-effect relationship.

What is fascinating is that this lunar influence on sleep exists even in urban settings with significant light pollution, suggesting an innate biological rhythm synchronized with the moon. This adds to the mounting evidence showing that our natural sleep-wake cycles are influenced by many factors beyond just sunrise and sunset (Cleveland Clinic, 2021).

A Sleep-Wake Cycle Overview

As the last crimson rays of sunlight slipped beyond the horizon, painting the sky in hues of orange and purple, Lando found himself in the small town where he grew up. It was a place nestled amidst rolling hills and surrounded by the serenity of nature. The world around him began to wrap itself in the comforting blanket of darkness, signaling the beginning of a magical sequence known as the sleep-wake cycle.

Lando, a curious and introspective soul, always found solace in observing the rhythms of life. As night descended upon the town, he took a moment to step outside and breathe in the cool evening air. The stars twinkled above, casting a gentle glow on the landscape. In this quiet moment, he felt an inexplicable connection to a larger, unseen ballet unfolding across the globe.

In his mind's eye, Lando pictured a street vendor in bustling Bangkok, skillfully packing away his wares as darkness settled in. He imagined a farmer in the vast plains of Kansas, finally surrendering to sleep beneath the vast expanse of twinkling stars. And in Rome, he envisioned a writer awakening with the first rays of dawn, feeling a surge of fresh inspiration.

Although separated by miles and cultures, they were all intertwined in the same global rhythm of rest and wakefulness. Lando marveled at the intricate dance orchestrated by the sleep-wake cycle, a 24-hour internal clock choreographed by nature itself. The conductor of this symphony was the suprachiasmatic nucleus, a group of cells nestled within the depths of the brain's hypothalamus.

Under the command of this maestro, Lando understood that our bodies ebb and flow through states of alertness and drowsiness, guided by the shifting scales of light and darkness. During the vibrant daylight hours, his body experienced the high tide of wakefulness, fueled by the hormone cortisol. The world brimmed with energy as people in bustling cities and tranquil landscapes carried out their daily routines.

But as evening descended and shadows lengthened, the delicate hormone melatonin began its ascent. Lando imagined the moon casting a soft, silvery glow over different corners of the globe. From the grand old city of London to the quiet hamlets of rural China, bodies succumbed to the embrace of rest. Muscles relaxed, breathing slowed, and thoughts drifted away as they entered the sleep domain.

Lando recognized that healing and restoration took place in this mysterious and essential part of the cycle. It was a land of dreams, where memories were sorted, the day's learning was consolidated, and the body found rejuvenation. And as the dawn broke, from the towering skyscrapers of New York to the rustic countryside of India, beings awakened refreshed, ready to engage in the dance of a new day.

In this personal journey of observing the sleep-wake cycle, Lando realized it was more than a biological necessity. It was a testament to the shared human experience, a rhythm transcending borders, cultures, and languages. It was a dance choreographed by Nature, uniting people across the globe in a collective production of rest and wakefulness.

As Lando lay down to sleep that night, he felt a sense of awe and gratitude for his place in this age-old dance. He knew that wherever he found himself in the world, he was part of this larger tapestry of life. And as he closed his eyes, he whispered a silent appreciation for the intricate workings of the sleep-wake cycle, knowing that it would guide him through the night and gently awaken him to a brand new day.

But how exactly does this process regulate our sleeping patterns?

How the Sleep-Wake Cycle Regulates Sleep Patterns

The symphony of the sleep-wake cycle resounds across the globe, uniting humanity in a shared rhythm. Whether it is a baby in Rio, a teenager in Tokyo, or an elderly gentleman in Nairobi, the cycle regulates our sleep patterns, influencing our slumbers and wakefulness.

From the moment we are born, the sleep-wake process begins its lifelong role as the conductor of our rest. A newborn in the vibrant city of Rio de Janeiro may sleep as much as 16 hours a day, scattered randomly throughout the 24 hours. This pattern reflects the immature sleep-wake cycle, which gradually aligns with the rhythm of day and night as the baby grows.

Fast forward to the bustling metropolis of Tokyo, where a teenager battles against a sleep-wake cycle shifted toward late nights and late mornings—a phenomenon called the phase delay. Despite societal demands, the adolescent's internal clock pushes for later sleep times, a challenge teens face globally. Understanding this natural shift can inform school schedules and social expectations, aiding teenagers in achieving their sleep requirements.

Now, envision an older adult in South Africa, waking before dawn. With age, the sleep-wake process often advances, leading to earlier sleep and wake times, known as the phase advance. While societal norms may accommodate these shifts, it is essential to ensure older people get sufficient quality sleep, as it plays a critical role in maintaining cognitive functions and overall health.

The sleep-wake cycle also influences the structure of our sleep. Imagine an artist in Paris, lost in dreams during the early night. This is the realm of REM sleep, a phase abundant in the first sleep cycles and crucial for memory consolidation and emotional regulation. Later in the night, the artist experiences more non-REM sleep, which is vital for physical restoration.

Whether you are a parent in Sydney trying to synchronize with your newborn's sleep, a college student in Mumbai grappling with late-night study sessions, or a retiree in Moscow enjoying the tranquility of early mornings, understanding your sleep-wake cycle can help. Acknowledging its influence can lead to better sleep habits, improved health, and enhanced well-being.

Remember, the sleep-wake process is not a soloist but an orchestra, with each component playing a crucial role.

Unpacking Circadian Rhythms

Take a moment and consider this: As you hustle through your day, an invisible rhythm guides you, an innate biological drumbeat. It dictates when you feel awake, drowsiness creeps in, and even when your hunger strikes. Your circadian rhythm is your personal 24-hour internal clock, operating in the background to coordinate a symphony of bodily functions.

It is fascinating that "circadian" originates from the Latin words "circa," implying "around," and "diem," indicating "day." Fittingly, these rhythms orchestrate our biology and behavior around the earth's daily rotation. Every living being, from the smallest bacterium to the enormous blue whale, dances to the beat of this circadian metronome.

You might wonder, where is the conductor of this grand orchestra? The answer lies within your brain, in a small region called the suprachiasmatic nucleus, or the SCN. Located in the hypothalamus, this cluster of nerve cells responds to light cues, primarily sunlight, to regulate the circadian rhythm.

What is astonishing is how the circadian rhythm influences various physiological processes. For instance, a study found that the disruption of circadian rhythms could lead to an increased risk of mood disorders, decreased well-being, and cognitive functions (Bechtel, 2015).

Moreover, the circadian rhythm plays a substantial role in your sleep-wake cycle. Light exposure, particularly the blue light emitted from electronic devices, can throw this cycle off balance, leading to sleep issues such as insomnia or daytime sleepiness (Newsom, 2020).

But it does not stop at sleep. Your circadian rhythm also regulates hormone production, feeding patterns, body temperature, and even cell regeneration. A study published suggests that circadian misalignment can adversely affect metabolism and body weight regulation, providing a potential link to obesity (Chaput et al., 2022).

While these rhythms are endogenous, meaning they originate within us, they can be influenced by external cues like light, temperature, and meal times. Harnessing these cues to align with our circadian rhythm can promote health and well-being, a concept utilized in therapies like light therapy for seasonal affective disorder or jet lag management.

In essence, understanding your circadian rhythm is like decrypting a secret language of your body. As you learn to listen to this rhythm, you are one step closer to embracing a healthier, more harmonious lifestyle. This inner rhythm, it seems, is not just a scientific curiosity; it is a fundamental part of who we are.

How Circadian Rhythms Influence Sleep and Wakefulness

Understanding the rhythm of life involves deciphering your circadian rhythm and its remarkable influence on sleep and wakefulness. This 24-hour internal clock, as we have discussed earlier, operates behind the scenes and guides your daily dance between alertness and drowsiness, forming a vital element in regulating and maintaining overall health and well-being.

The circadian rhythm's impact on sleep becomes apparent when you think about the sudden afternoon fatigue or the alertness that peaks in the evening. These are not random fluctuations but events carefully orchestrated by your circadian rhythm, following the beat of your internal clock.

At the heart of this rhythm is the SCN. The SCN responds to light—particularly sunlight—and sends signals to numerous brain parts, including the pineal gland, which adjusts the production of melatonin. During the day, melatonin levels are low, keeping you alert, but as night falls and light diminishes, melatonin production ramps up, ushering in the call to sleep.

However, the influence of the circadian rhythm extends beyond merely controlling sleep and wakefulness. A study suggests that the circadian rhythm regulates sleep timing, quantity, and quality (Goel et al., 2013).

This regulation ensures that sleep stages unfold optimally, providing the rejuvenation your body and mind need.

While the circadian rhythm is an internal system, it is not immune to external influences. Light exposure, meal timing, and physical activity can shift this rhythm. In one published study, researchers found that disruptions to the circadian rhythm, such as those caused by shift work or jet lag, can lead to sleep disorders, mental health issues, and metabolic problems (Walker et al., 2020).

Aligning your lifestyle with your circadian rhythm is vital to ensuring healthy sleep patterns and optimal alertness during waking hours. Simple strategies, like getting ample sunlight during the day, keeping a consistent sleep schedule, and limiting light exposure in the evening, can help anchor your sleep-wake cycle and enhance your overall health.

In its silent, persistent ticking, the circadian rhythm embodies a pearl of profound wisdom—the understanding of time and how to best synchronize with the world around us. It is a dance of biology, environment, and lifestyle, where mastering the steps can lead to optimal sleep, daytime alertness, and other benefits.

The Suprachiasmatic Nucleus's Role in the Brain

Nestled within the hypothalamus, this tiny but mighty collection of neurons steers the ship of our circadian rhythms, guiding the tides of our sleep-wake cycle and numerous other physiological processes.

Let me simplify this complex machinery with a helpful analogy. Imagine a bustling city. Just as a city has a central hub governing and regulating the rhythm of life, the SCN serves the same purpose for our bodies. It acts as the main clock, setting the tempo for mini peripheral clocks throughout the body. As the central hub, the SCN ensures harmonious synchrony, maintaining the alignment of the body's biological functions.

What influences this hub? The SCN responds primarily to light cues. Light penetrates your eyes each morning and travels along the optic nerves, signaling the SCN that a new day has dawned.

In turn, the SCN kick-starts your day, setting off a cascade of biological processes to prepare your body for wakefulness. It signals the pineal gland to halt the production of melatonin, resulting in increased alertness.

But the SCN's role extends beyond daylight hours. As evening sets in and light decreases, the SCN communicates the onset of darkness, triggering the pineal gland to increase melatonin production, guiding your body into sleep mode.

Yet, the SCN's impact goes even further. It influences core body temperature, hunger, hormonal release, and even mood. It is a silent, relentless engine, working 24/7 to keep our internal world in order.

Synchronization with the SCN is vital for health and well-being. Desynchrony, like that experienced by shift workers or frequent flyers, can lead to sleep disorders, mental health issues, or metabolic problems. Therefore, understanding and respecting the SCN's role and our body's rhythm is critical.

In conclusion, the SCN, the brain's unseen maestro, masterfully conducts the symphony of our physiological functions, affirming that life operates on rhythms and cycles. Just as a city never truly sleeps but constantly hums with energy, so too do our bodies, regulated by the tireless SCN, strive for balance in the rhythm of life. Thus, the SCN proves to be not just a part of our brain but an essential hub that helps us navigate the dance between night and day, sleep and wakefulness, and rest and activity.

The Suprachiasmatic Nucleus' Control Over the Sleep-Wake Cycle

Ah! Yes! The daily dance between sleep and wakefulness. Unseen, yet ever-present. Imagine it as an artist, painting our days with hues of energy and our nights with strokes of rest.

The SCN is like the DJ of your brain, mixing tracks of light signals and internal cues to compose your 24-hour rhythm. When dawn breaks, rays of sunlight creep into your eyes, subtly informing your SCN that it is time to start the party. It responds by dialing up the "wakefulness" track, ushering in alertness, focus, and vitality.

It does this by activating a network of neural connections that stimulate various parts of the brain and body. Hormones like cortisol flood your system, kick-starting your metabolism and energy levels. Your body temperature rises, priming your muscles for movement. Meanwhile, your brain waves quicken, tuning in to the world around you.

As day turns to dusk, the SCN starts to remix the rhythm. The dwindling light tells it that it is time to mellow things down. So it gradually lowers the volume on the "wakefulness" track and smoothly transitions to the soothing "sleep" melody.

Your body temperature cools, muscles relax, and brain waves slow. Hormones like melatonin begin their nightly serenade, lulling you into a peaceful slumber. In this manner, the SCN ensures you get the rest you need right on cue.

Yet, the SCN's influence extends beyond mere sleep and wakefulness. It also coordinates other biological rhythms, like hunger and hormone release, tuning them into the same 24-hour cycle. This seamless integration helps maintain balance and harmony in our bodies.

Intriguingly, your SCN does not work solo. It engages in a constant feedback loop with your body and environment, adapting your sleep-wake cycle to changing conditions. A long day at work, a late-night snack, or a shift in time zones can tweak the SCN's playlist, altering your sleep-wake rhythm.

With the SCN in the mix, you are not just responding to the world; you are dancing to your own unique beat. And that, in essence, is the true magic of the SCN's control over your sleep-wake cycle. An intricate dance between light, time, and biology, all choreographed to the rhythm of life.

Factors That Influence the Sleep-Wake Cycle and Fixing Them

The harmony of our sleep-wake cycle, a seamless dance of light and dark, waking and resting, can often be disrupted. But what rogue elements step on our rhythmic toes, and how can we get our dance back in sync? Here are some key factors and everyday solutions to get us twirling to the rhythm of life again.

- **Light Exposure:** As our sleep maestro, the SCN responds to changes in light, adjusting our sleep-wake rhythms accordingly. But artificial light, moreover blue light screens, can confuse our natural rhythm.

  Solution: Reduce screen time in the evening. Try adopting a "lights-out" rule an hour before bed, giving your body the signal that it is time to wind down. Make this a fun routine for kids with story-telling sessions or drawing in the dim light.

- **Diet and Meal Timing:** Our sleep rhythm and metabolism are intertwined. Heavy meals late at night or caffeine can disrupt sleep.

<u>**Solution:**</u> Try having dinner a few hours before bed and limit caffeine intake after midafternoon. For teenagers who love late-night snacks and energy drinks, try introducing healthier evening snacks, like nuts or fruits.

- **Physical Activity:** Regular exercise promotes healthy sleep. However, intense exercise close to bedtime can disrupt the sleep cycle.

  <u>**Solution:**</u> Schedule exercise for the morning or afternoon. Encourage children to play outside during the day, while adults can slot in a brisk lunchtime walk or a postwork meditation session.

- **Stress:** Anxiety, worry, and high stress levels can interfere with the sleep-wake cycle.

  <u>**Solution:**</u> Develop a calming bedtime routine with relaxation techniques such as reading or a warm bubble bath. Encourage teenagers to journal their thoughts before bedtime as a way of offloading stress.

- **Age:** Our sleep patterns change as we age. Teens tend to be night owls, while adults may wake early.

  <u>**Solution:**</u> For adolescents, allow for later wake-up times when possible, and ensure they catch up on sleep during weekends. For seniors, a short afternoon nap can compensate for early rising, but keep it brief to avoid disrupting nighttime sleep.

By understanding these factors, we can choreograph our sleep-wake dance to our own beat, improving our sleep and our daytime energy levels, mood, and overall health. Remember, it is a personal journey, and what works best will vary from person to person.

Get ready to unlock the secrets of restful slumber with my transformative sleep methods, your guide to rejuvenation and achieving peak daytime performance.

Sleep Remedy One: Sunset Visualization Technique

Find a cozy posture, sitting or reclining, and paint a serene sunset in your mind's eye. Envision the vivid hues, soft wind, and tranquil atmosphere. Concentrate on the slow shift from day to twilight, easing yourself into a state of relaxation and sleep preparedness.

Sleep Remedy Two: Chamomile Tea for Restful Sleep

Immerse a teaspoon of desiccated chamomile flowers in a mug of steaming water for a duration of five to 10 minutes. Strain the infusion and, if you prefer, enhance its sweetness with honey. Alternatively, you can steep 1 chamomile tea bag in hot water. Sip this soothing concoction half an hour prior to retiring for the night to help synchronize your sleep-wake rhythm and foster a sense of tranquility.

Bonus Remedy: You can also try mixing in a teaspoon of magnesium powder until it seamlessly melds into the solution.

On to melatonin we go.

Chapter 3:

Melatonin's Role: Tapping Into the Sleep Hormone

Miraculous melatonin should shower some melatonin to the eyes so that eyes can kiss the dreams during sleep. –Dr. Sreeremya

As dusk settles, a quiet hormone named melatonin begins its nocturnal serenade, lulling the body into a peaceful slumber. This chapter explores melatonin's dance with sleep, guiding us through the moonlit pathways where biology merges with the realm of dreams. Ready yourself for an illuminating journey into the intimate relationship between this humble hormone and the enigmatic world of sleep.

An Introduction to Melatonin

Regarding our biological rhythm, few molecules command the respect accorded to melatonin, the night-bringer and guardian of our nightly slumber. This hormone, secreted primarily by the pineal gland nestled deep within our brains, has an almost mythical status in our understanding of the human sleep cycle. The intimate relationship between melatonin and sleep has been the focus of extensive research. Yet, it continues to fascinate scientists and laypeople alike with its intricate operations and profound impacts.

Melatonin's role begins as the sky darkens and the bustle of the day gradually subsides. Its rise in our bloodstream is a signal, a gentle whisper that it is time to wind down and prepare for rest. But melatonin is not just a simple chemical switch. From lowering body temperature to slowing metabolic processes, the effects of this hormone pervade our physical being, easing us into the regenerative embrace of sleep.

However, melatonin's influence extends beyond the realm of sleep. It is known to be a potent antioxidant, and evidence suggests a potential role in immunity and aging processes. It is also critical in regulating other hormones, underlining its central position in our complex biological systems.

Moreover, melatonin production is intimately tied to our environment's cycle of light and darkness. It is our body's way of keeping time, aligning our internal rhythms with the Earth's rotation. This synchronization has far-reaching implications for our physical and mental health, and disruptions can lead to sleep disorders and associated health complications.

Our understanding of melatonin is still a work in progress despite its crucial importance. The hormone's complex interactions within our bodies, its relationship with light exposure, and the precise mechanisms by which it influences sleep are subjects of ongoing research.

This humble hormone's role in our sleep-wake cycle is a fascinating testament to the intricate design of human biology. As we peel back the layers of scientific understanding, melatonin reveals its depth and complexity, solidifying its position as an extraordinary part of our biological makeup. We invite you on a journey into the captivating world of melatonin, where the domains of science and slumber intersect, offering profound insights into the silent, curious dance of sleep.

The Importance of Melatonin in Regulating Sleep-Wake Cycles

As we have recently learned, melatonin is a hormone mainly created in our brains' pineal glands. It performs a critical role in regulating our sleep-wake cycles. Its importance emerges as the curtain of daylight falls, and its secretion in our bodies increases, signaling that it is time to rest.

Earlier, we also established melatonin's release into our system follows the circadian rhythm, which mirrors the natural cycle of light and dark. This rhythm ensures we are awake during the day and sleeping at night. Melatonin plays a pivotal role in governing this rhythm. As light levels drop, melatonin production ramps up, guiding us toward sleep. When dawn breaks, melatonin production decreases, allowing us to awaken.

The function of melatonin is not merely sleep induction, though. It's a crucial component in setting that internal biological clock we discussed in the previous chapter by aligning our bodily functions with the daily rhythm. For instance, as melatonin prepares us for sleep, it also influences various other bodily functions.

Beyond its impact on sleep, melatonin is relevant in other health areas. Did you know it is also an antioxidant, protecting our cells from damage? Recent research also suggests a role for melatonin in modulating immune responses. These additional roles illustrate how interconnected melatonin is with various aspects of our health.

However, our modern lifestyle often disrupts the natural tides of melatonin production. These disruptions can lead to various sleep disorders and other health issues.

Therefore, understanding and respecting the role of melatonin in our lives is essential for optimal health. By aligning our lifestyle habits with our natural circadian rhythm—dimming lights in the evening, limiting screen time before bed, and maintaining regular sleep and wake times—we can support melatonin production and improve sleep quality.

In conclusion, melatonin is more than just a sleep hormone. It is a crucial element of our body's rhythm, key in aligning our internal processes with the outside world. This journey into the world of melatonin underscores the importance of this hormone in our daily lives. It emphasizes the need for a lifestyle that respects our natural sleep-wake cycles.

Did You Know?

Your sense of smell diminishes when you are asleep. Unlike hearing and touch, which remain alert to our surroundings even in slumber, our olfactory system takes a break during sleep.

This fascinating phenomenon is thought to occur due to the brain's selective disengagement from sensory inputs during sleep. While we sleep, especially during REM sleep, the brain merges memories and processes information from the day. To accomplish this effectively, it reduces the distraction from sensory inputs.

The thalamus, a brain component, acts as a relay station for sensory information and is known to reduce the transmission of most sensory signals to the brain's cortex during sleep. The olfactory system, however, bypasses the thalamus, suggesting that other mechanisms might be at play during the reduction in smell sensitivity.

One theory suggests that the olfactory bulb (the first brain region to receive signals about odors) might enter a state of inactivity during sleep, effectively reducing our ability to detect smells. However, more research is needed to understand these mechanisms fully.

Conversely, it is interesting to note that not all smells are ignored. Studies have found that certain scents, particularly those associated with danger like smoke or gas, can rouse us from sleep, hinting at a potential survival mechanism (feather&black, n.d.).

The Pineal Gland

Deep within the folds of the human brain lies the pineal gland, a tiny, pea-sized organ that, despite its size, plays an indispensable role in our biological systems. Often referred to as the "third eye," this small yet mighty gland has intrigued scientists and philosophers alike, and understanding its function unveils a fascinating facet of human physiology.

The pineal gland's claim to fame is its role as the primary producer of melatonin, the hormone critical for regulating our sleep-wake cycles. Like a diligent factory working in harmony with the outside world, the pineal gland responds to changing light conditions, churning out melatonin as darkness descends. With this rise in melatonin levels, the body gets the signal to prepare for sleep, initiating a cascade of physiological changes that foster rest and rejuvenation.

But the pineal gland's responsibility extends beyond sleep regulation. Its influence seeps into various facets of our well-being. For instance, it helps modulate our mood and plays a part in our body's ability to manage stress. The gland's function is complex and multi-layered, each role interlinking with another, much like a meticulously arranged domino setup.

Moreover, the pineal gland's interaction with light and darkness underscores its role in connecting us with our environment. As the sun sets, the absence of light prompts the pineal gland to step up melatonin production, linking our internal processes with the external world in a dance as old as time itself. This harmony is essential to our overall health, with disruptions potentially leading to sleep disorders, mood changes, and more.

One challenge facing our modern lifestyle is artificial light. This constant illumination can confuse the pineal gland, disrupting melatonin production and our sleep-wake cycles. Therefore, understanding the workings of the pineal gland offers a pathway to better sleep hygiene and improved health.

The Changes in Melatonin Levels During Day and Night

Daytime

As the sun climbs across the sky, the world awakens to the rhythm of life. Humans, too, fueled by the bustling energy of daylight, engage in their daily activities. But beneath this vibrancy, in the sanctuary of our brains, the pineal gland adopts a quieter role. During the day, our melatonin levels remain at their lowest. This small yet significant hormone takes a backseat, allowing other biochemical actors to enter the limelight. Cortisol, the "stress hormone," gets its turn to peak, fostering alertness and focus, while melatonin retreats, laying low in the backdrop.

Just as a library quiets down when students are in study mode, the pineal gland slows down melatonin production during the day. It is as though our internal system understands that it is time for activity, not sleep. This reduction in melatonin assists in maintaining our wakefulness, allowing us to go about our day unencumbered by the call of slumber. It is a testament to the intricate chemical balance governing our biological rhythms, ensuring we are in sync with the world.

Nighttime

As the sun dips below the horizon and twilight yields to the night, a shift occurs within our bodies. The pineal gland springs into action after lying dormant during the daylight hours. Melatonin production kicks up a notch, like a bakery preparing for the day ahead in the early hours, churning out fresh loaves of sleep-inducing hormones. As melatonin levels rise, our bodies receive the signal that it's time to slow down, wind down, and prepare for sleep.

This increase in melatonin production is the body's natural response to darkness, a biological process that dates back to our ancestors. It is akin to flipping a switch, but instead of turning off lights, it dims our consciousness, leading us gently toward the restorative domains of sleep.

However, this shift is not a blunt on-and-off process. It is more like a gentle gradient, a subtle transition that varies among individuals and can be influenced by various factors, such as age, lifestyle, and exposure to light. Understanding this nocturnal melatonin surge gives us a unique perspective on the journey toward sleep and the biological processes that guide us there.

The Impact of Light Exposure on Melatonin Production

In the grand theater of human biology, Charlotte stood as an eager spectator, ready to witness the delicate dance between light and melatonin. She imagined herself stepping into the spotlight, playing the role of an enthusiastic observer, as the performance unfolded, intricately dictating the rhythm of her sleep-wake cycle.

As the sun began its ascent, casting a golden glow across the world, Charlotte felt the stirrings of energy within her. Her body responded to the daylight, awakening to the promise of a new day. Within the depths of her brain, the pineal gland, a tiny organ responsible for melatonin production, acknowledged this signal. It respected the flood of light, slowing down melatonin production to keep hormone levels low throughout the day. It was as if the teacher in a classroom maintained silence, allowing students to concentrate and remain alert.

But as the daylight slowly retreated, making way for the curtain of nightfall, the performance took a different turn. Darkness enveloped the world, and the stage was set for melatonin to play its starring role. The pineal gland shifted gears, sensing the absence of light, and increased melatonin production like a well-timed stage cue. This surge of hormones served as a gentle nod, guiding Charlotte's body toward the restful embrace of sleep.

However, the advent of artificial light disrupted this age-old performance. Charlotte witnessed the pervasive glow of screens and indoor lighting, casting a constant spotlight that overshadowed the pineal gland's cues. It caused delays or reductions in melatonin production, preventing the hormone from taking its nightly bow. The disruption of light-induced melatonin suppression resulted in difficulties falling asleep or experiencing fragmented sleep.

Charlotte learned that not all light impacts melatonin production equally. Blue light, abundant in digital screens, had a powerful influence on suppressing melatonin. It was like an unruly audience member causing disruptions, making it difficult for melatonin to perform its role effectively.

With this newfound knowledge, Charlotte recognized the need to adapt her behaviors to support her melatonin production. She consciously tried to limit her evening screen time, allowing herself to disconnect from the digital world. She discovered software that reduced blue light exposure, creating a more favorable environment for her body's natural rhythms. Charlotte also cultivated a sleep-friendly space, creating a sanctuary where she could find solace and rest.

Understanding the profound impact of light on melatonin production deepened Charlotte's appreciation for her connection with nature's rhythms. It served as a reminder of the delicate balance she needed to strike with her modern lifestyle. Charlotte marveled at light's profound influence on her sleep health, vowing to prioritize the harmony between light and melatonin to achieve restful nights and embrace the gift of rejuvenating sleep.

Natural Ways to Boost Melatonin Levels

As previously discussed, melatonin is crucial in regulating our sleep-wake cycle. While melatonin supplements are available, natural ways to boost its production within our bodies exist. By making certain lifestyle adjustments and harnessing the power of our environment, we can promote the biological synthesis of melatonin.

One key factor in melatonin production is exposure to light. Our bodies respond to light cues, with darkness triggering the release of melatonin. Creating a conducive environment for sleep is essential to enhance natural melatonin production. Dimming the lights in the evening signals to our bodies that it is time to wind down. Avoiding exposure to bright screens, such as those from electronic devices, is crucial. Instead, engaging in activities such as eating tryptophan-rich foods (pumpkins, peanuts, fish, etc.) and banishing screens from the bedroom can help promote the natural release of melatonin.

Another factor to consider is our sleep schedule. Maintaining a consistent sleep routine reinforces our body's internal clock and supports the natural production of melatonin. Going to sleep and waking up at the same time daily helps regulate our sleep-wake cycle, optimizing melatonin synthesis. Exposure to natural light during the day also aids in this process. Spending time outdoors, especially in the morning, exposes us to sunlight and reinforces our body's melatonin production patterns.

Furthermore, our dietary choices can influence melatonin production. Certain foods contain naturally occurring compounds that support their synthesis. Tart cherries, for instance, are a rich source of melatonin. Consuming tart cherry juice or incorporating these cherries into our diet can help boost melatonin levels. Other foods, such as bananas, oats, and nuts, contain nutrients that contribute to melatonin production.

Additionally, creating a sleep-friendly environment is essential. Make sure your bedroom is cool, dark, and quiet to promote restful sleep. Investing in blackout curtains or wearing an eye mask can help eliminate sources of light that disrupt melatonin production. Managing stress levels through relaxation techniques, guided imagery (concentrating on positive images), or autogenic training (promoting calm feelings) can also improve sleep quality and support natural melatonin synthesis.

Did You Know?

Sleeping at high altitudes can indeed affect your sleep quality. At elevations above 13,200 feet (4,000 meters), oxygen levels start to decrease significantly. This scarcity of oxygen, also known as hypoxia, can disrupt your sleep in several ways.

Firstly, hypoxia can lead to a condition known as periodic breathing during sleep. This is characterized by cycles of normal breathing, followed by a decrease or complete cessation of breathing, causing frequent awakenings. As a result, people at high altitudes often experience increased sleep fragmentation, leading to poor sleep quality.

Secondly, hypoxia can lead to more time spent in lighter stages of sleep and less time in restorative REM sleep. This shift in sleep architecture contributes to the feelings of sleepiness and fatigue that people often report at high altitudes.

Finally, sleeping at high altitudes can increase the frequency of nocturnal awakenings due to the need to urinate, a condition known as nocturia. This is due to increased urinary output caused by the body's response to hypoxia.

In response to these challenges, the human body can acclimate over time (usually a few days to weeks) to handle the lower oxygen levels, which can improve sleep quality at high altitudes. However, the process and speed of acclimatization can vary greatly between individuals (feather&black, n.d.).

Using Melatonin Supplements as Sleeping Aids

Melatonin supplements have gained popularity as a sleep aid but like any intervention, they have pros and cons. Understanding melatonin supplements' potential benefits and drawbacks can help individuals make informed decisions about their sleep health.

One of the main advantages of melatonin supplements is their ability to regulate sleep-wake cycles. For those struggling with jet lag or shift work, melatonin supplements can help adjust sleep patterns and promote faster adaptation to new schedules. They can also benefit individuals with delayed sleep phase syndrome or other circadian rhythm disorders, providing a way to synchronize their internal clock with the desired sleep schedule.

Another advantage is that melatonin supplements are generally considered safe and well-tolerated when used appropriately. They are available over-the-counter in many countries and are nonaddictive, making them a preferred choice for individuals seeking a short-term sleep aid without the risk of dependency. Additionally, melatonin supplements have a relatively short half-life, allowing users to wake up feeling refreshed without residual drowsiness.

However, there are certain cons to consider when using melatonin supplements. One concern is the potential for side effects. While uncommon, some individuals may experience daytime drowsiness, headaches, or dizziness after taking melatonin. It is recommended to start on a lower dose and gradually increase if needed, under the advice of a medical practitioner, to minimize the risk of adverse effects.

Another aspect to be aware of is the potential for interactions with other medications. Melatonin has certain drug interactions, such as with blood thinners, immunosuppressants, and sedatives. It is vital to consult a medical practitioner before initiating melatonin supplementation to ensure it does not interfere with existing medications or underlying health conditions.

Furthermore, melatonin supplements may not be suitable for everyone. Pregnant or breastfeeding women, individuals with certain medical conditions, and those taking specific medications should exercise caution and seek medical advice before using melatonin supplements. It is essential to consider individual circumstances and consult a healthcare professional to determine the appropriateness of melatonin supplementation.

Lastly, it is worth noting that melatonin supplements may not address the underlying causes of sleep difficulties. While they can effectively manage certain sleep disorders or temporary disruptions, they do not replace healthy sleep habits and a conducive sleep environment. Establishing a consistent sleep routine, practicing good sleep hygiene, and addressing any underlying issues contributing to sleep disturbances is crucial for long-term sleep health.

In conclusion, melatonin supplements offer potential benefits in regulating sleep-wake cycles and can be helpful for specific sleep disorders or situations. They are generally safe and nonaddictive when used correctly. However, possible side effects, medication interactions, and the need for individual suitability should be considered.

Embrace the methods below for a serene journey into relaxation, intertwining mindfulness, breathwork, and gentle movements to usher profound, rejuvenating rest. Your best sleep awaits when trying out one of my sleeping remedies below.

Sleep Remedy One: Magnesium-Rich Banana Smoothie

Blend together 1 ripe banana, 1 cup of almond milk, 1 tablespoon of almond butter, and a handful of spinach. Add 1 teaspoon of magnesium powder for an extra boost. Enjoy this smoothie in the evening to promote melatonin production and a restful sleep

Sleep Remedy Two: Oatmeal with Banana and Honey

Cook ½ cup oats with 1 cup water or milk. Top with sliced ½ banana and drizzle with 1 teaspoon honey. Enjoy as a calming bedtime bowl. Oats are rich in complex carbohydrates and contain nutrients like vitamin B6, which supports the conversion of tryptophan into serotonin. Bananas provide vitamin B6 and natural sugars, while honey offers a touch of sweetness for a comforting bedtime snack.

Get excited because the next stop in our journey to better sleep is about creating your ideal sleeping space. I can't wait to share my insights with you.

Chapter 4:

Designing Your Ideal Sleep Haven

Nothing makes you feel better than when you get into a hotel bed, and the sheets feel so good. Why shouldn't you wake up like that every day? Spend money on your mattress and bedding because these things make a difference in your sleep and, ultimately, your happiness. –Bobby Berk

Step into the domain of creating your dream sleeping space. This chapter unfurls the secrets to crafting a haven of tranquility tailored to your unique tastes. We will explore the essential elements that promote peaceful slumber, using techniques geared to soothe the senses to the perfect balance of comfort and functionality. Be prepared to reimagine your bedroom as an exquisite sleep oasis, expertly designed to usher in a profound, refreshing nightly rest.

The Importance of a Sleep-Conducive Environment

Lewis, our protagonist, found himself locked in a tussle with the elusive entity known as sleep. The dancing shadows of insomnia cavorted in his mind each night, spinning tales of fatigue, frustration, and far too many groggy mornings. With each sunrise, the lack of rest grew more potent, plaguing his daily life like an incessant echo in his tired mind.

Lewis couldn't escape the specter of sleeplessness. It stalked him in his waking hours, gnawing at his productivity, clouding his thoughts with an ever-thickening fog. Friends noted his unusual silence, his once vivacious energy replaced with all-consuming fatigue. His hobbies lay neglected, as did his dreams of writing a novel. Even the simplest tasks seemed insurmountable as lethargy overpowered ambition.

One particularly sleepless night, Lewis stumbled upon an article that claimed the power to transform his turmoil. It sang the praises of personalized bedroom design, arguing that our sleeping spaces should echo our preferences in aesthetics and comfort. It proposed ambient noise as an unseen lullaby, soothing the senses into tranquility. The promise was tempting, the potential relief palpable.

The following morning, worn from another restless night, Lewis embarked on his mission. He filled his room with elements that ignited his joy—books piled on antique tables, walls adorned with artwork mirrored his heart's yearning. Soft, muted tones replaced harsh hues, casting a soothing tranquility that beckoned slumber. For ambient noise, he selected the gentle whispers of distant waves, a lullaby that harked back to carefree childhood holidays on sun-drenched beaches.

Night fell, casting a shroud of stars against the velvety sky. Lewis, lying in the comforting embrace of his newly designed sanctuary, listened as the murmur of waves washed over him. His heart, usually racing with anticipation of the struggle, quieted. His mind, ever eager to spin tales of tomorrow, stilled.

Sleep, once a torturous tease, tiptoed in through the soft symphony of his serene surroundings. It danced in the glow of the moonlight filtering through the curtains and kissed away the shadows of insomnia that had held Lewis captive. Lewis surrendered to the sweet embrace of undisturbed sleep for the first time in months.

And thus, in a room designed to echo his heart's whispers amidst the gentle susurration of distant waves, Lewis found his respite, sanctuary, and ticket to the dreamland he had sorely missed. His struggle with sleeplessness began to soften, one serene night at a time.

But how did he and so many others manage to fix the problem? Let us take another journey.

Did You Know?

Contrary to common belief, no person sleeps straight through the night. It is normal for everyone to experience brief awakenings, even if we are unaware of them. These awakenings, or arousals, are a part of our sleep cycle and occur as we transition between different sleep stages, especially REM and NREM sleep.

We cycle through these stages roughly every 90 minutes during a typical night. When a cycle ends, we have a brief period of semi-awake time, which most people do not remember in the morning. This process is normal and does not necessarily mean your sleep is of poor quality.

However, if these arousals become more prolonged or more frequent, they can become disruptive and lead to feelings of unrefreshed sleep or insomnia. Factors such as stress, sleep disorders (like sleep apnea), alcohol, certain medications, or poor sleep hygiene can increase the frequency and length of these awakenings (feather&black, n.d.).

The Sanctum of the Bedroom

The bedroom is a sanctum—a retreat designed to encapsulate tranquility and peace. A place where the din of daily life falls away, replaced by the hushed whispers of dreams waiting to unfurl. The environment we cultivate within this sanctuary profoundly impacts our sleep, our health, and, indeed, our lives.

With careful consideration of comfort, noise levels, lighting, and temperature, we can design a space that genuinely promotes restful sleep.

Comfort

Sophia's love for the visually aesthetic often led her to make design choices that, while stunning, didn't necessarily prioritize comfort. Her beautiful but rock-hard mattress and minimalistic, neck-twisting pillows were a testament to this. When Sophia finally prioritized comfort, she was astonished by the change.

She chose a mattress tailored to her sleeping style, a down-filled duvet, and supportive pillows that cradled her neck as she slept. The tactile sensation of soft cotton sheets against her skin and the plush comfort under her body transformed her sleeping experience. Sophia learned that the significance of comfort in the bedroom could not be overstated, and it soon became her first rule of thumb in designing a space conducive to a restful night's sleep.

Noise Levels

Peter lived in a bustling city neighborhood where noise was as constant as the air he breathed. The urban cacophony of car horns, sirens, and voices flowed into his bedroom, disrupting his sleep. One day, he decided to combat the sleep thief with noise-canceling curtains and a white noise machine.

The curtains absorbed the din from outside while the white noise machine filled his bedroom with soothing sounds of rain, waves, or wind. The ambient noise created a bubble of tranquility in his room, muffling disruptive noises. Peter's story serves as a reminder that regulating noise levels is critical to creating a sleep-friendly environment.

Lighting

Alice was a night owl. The glow of her laptop often illuminated her room until the wee hours. Unbeknownst to her, the artificial light was messing with her body's internal clock, suppressing melatonin secretion.

Alice's journey to better sleep began when she replaced harsh lights with warm, dimmable ones and started using blackout curtains to block out unwanted light. She also implemented a digital sunset, switching off electronic devices an hour before sleep. Her new lighting regime reinforced her body's natural circadian rhythm, cueing it to wind down as the lights dimmed, encouraging a deeper, more restful sleep.

Temperature

Kevin often woke up in the middle of the night, either shivering or sweating. His sleep was a casualty of his disregard for room temperature. A quick Google search revealed that a cooler room temperature, around 65 degrees Fahrenheit (18.3 degrees Celsius), was more conducive to good sleep.

With this knowledge, Kevin adjusted his room temperature and improved his sleep drastically. He was no longer jolted awake by discomfort, and his dreams flowed uninterrupted. Kevin's story underscores the importance of maintaining an optimal temperature for quality sleep.

The dance between sleep and the environment we create in our bedrooms is intimate. It's a relationship that thrives on consideration and care and on understanding the subtle and not-so-subtle factors that can disrupt or encourage restful sleep. Sophia, Peter, Alice, and Kevin's experiences illustrate the dramatic effect our sleep environment can have on our overall well-being. They offer valuable lessons on transforming our sleep sanctuaries to create the perfect backdrop for our nightly voyage into the world of dreams.

Did You Know?

A new bed can potentially enhance the amount of sleep people get by up to an hour each night. This might sound surprising, but the quality of our bed directly impacts our sleep comfort and overall sleep quality.

A study by the Sleep Council indicated that switching from an uncomfortable bed to a new one resulted in an average increase of 42 minutes of sleep. But if the old mattress was inferior, the improvement extended to a whopping 60 minutes of extra sleep.

The main reason behind this change relates to enhanced comfort and support. A bed that offers better support can alleviate pain and stiffness, which are everyday sleep disruptors. Moreover, a bed with better temperature regulation can prevent night sweats, another factor that can disturb sleep.

New beds also tend to be free from allergens that may accumulate in older mattresses over time, like dust mites and bed bugs, which can cause allergic reactions and interrupt sleep. Lastly, the psychological aspect of having a new and comfortable place to sleep can also encourage better sleep patterns (feather&black, n.d.).

One particular technique I would like to dive into next is ambient (colored) noise for improved sleep.

Exploring the Power of Colored Noise for Sleep

As someone who has battled the restless monsters of sleepless nights, I understand the frustration of staring at the ceiling, yearning for sleep's gentle embrace. The snarl of city streets, the neighbor's late-night TV saga, or even the unsettling silence—

each has its way of stealing our precious rest. It was during one such battle, deep into the shadows of the night, that I discovered the enticement of "colored noise."

Imagine harnessing the power of the rhythmic sea, the soothing rustle of autumn leaves, or the soft patter of rain against your window—all within your bedroom, a melody to guide you into the empire of dreams. This is the beauty of colored noise. These ambient sounds come in a spectrum of "colors."

When I first invited these symphonies of sleep into my bedroom, I was skeptical. Yet, as the warm hum of brown noise filled the room, I felt my mind surrender its stubborn grasp on the day's concerns. The city's symphony faded into insignificance, replaced by this comforting lullaby. The more I integrated colored noise into my nights, the more I noticed an improvement in my sleep quality and, subsequently, in my daytime vitality and focus.

Exploring the world of colored noise is like curating a personal soundscape, a lullaby tuned to your unique needs. Join me as we dive deeper into this topic, unraveling the science behind the colors of noise and how they mask disruptive sounds and promote better, more restful sleep. Let us turn the key to a world where sleep is not a battle, but a welcoming retreat, guided by the soothing whispers of your chosen noise color.

But what are the different colored noises we can use for ambiance? Remember, everyone's perception and response to different noise colors might vary, so what works best will often be a matter of personal preference.

Noise Color	Description	How It Helps Sleep
Blue	Higher frequency noise, with intensity increasing as frequency increases. Similar to the hiss of spraying water.	The high-pitched hiss of blue noise can mask other high-frequency sounds, like alarms or sirens. It might be less soothing for some, but others find it effective for sleep.
Brown	Lower frequency noise, with intensity decreasing as frequency increases. Sounds like a deep, rolling roar.	The deeper, more mellow sounds of brown noise can be soothing and help to block out disruptive lower-frequency sounds like traffic noise.
Green	Emphasizes mid-frequency sounds. Often described as the sounds of nature, like rustling leaves or a gentle rain.	This "natural" noise is usually calming, and the familiar sounds can be comforting, helping you to relax and sleep. It is also effective at masking mid-frequency sounds, like conversation.
White	Contains all frequencies at equal intensity. Sounds like a consistent, high-pitched hiss.	Masks all external sounds with its wide-frequency coverage. Its consistency helps to create a steady audio environment, promoting uninterrupted sleep.

Experimenting with different colors of noise might reveal the perfect backdrop for your tranquil nights. Tune into the symphony that sings you to sleep the most effectively, and enjoy the serenity it brings to your rest.

But what are the differences between these colored noises? This quartet of performers often goes unnoticed in our sleeping symphonies, their concert a subtle, soothing undercurrent to our nightly repose. They each possess a unique character, a different story to tell. In our quest for a good night's sleep, understanding these musicians can be instrumental in composing our perfect lullaby.

White Noise

Our first performer is white noise, the omnipresent virtuoso. Imagine a pianist pressing down all keys simultaneously, creating a sonic collage that is as consistent as it is complete. That is white noise for you, a sound that contains all audible frequencies in equal measure, much like white light having all spectrum colors.

White noise has a fantastic talent for blocking out disruptions. Its steady, unchanging flow provides a sound barrier that effectively masks sudden, jarring noises—from the neighbor's barking dog to the abrupt honk of a car. On nights when disruptive sounds threaten to steal your sleep, white noise steps in like a reliable old friend; its consistent hum is a protective blanket against auditory intrusions.

Blue Noise

Next, we have blue noise, the soprano of our sleep concert. Blue noise emphasizes the high frequencies. It is the sound of water rushing from a showerhead or the sizzle of a frying pan. It is the top note in our sleep symphony, offering a higher-pitched, more airy sound than its counterparts.

Blue noise is particularly adept at masking high-frequency sounds. While it might sound a little harsher to some, for others, it is just the ticket to a restful night. It is all about personal preference, finding the notes that resonate with you.

Green Noise

In comes green noise, the nature-loving middle child. Often described as the sound of a gentle rain or rustling leaves, green noise focuses on mid-frequency sounds. It is like a forest melody being played out in your room—a steady downpour on a leafy canopy, a persistent, calming rustle.

Green noise has a soothing effect, evoking feelings of serenity and peace. It is like taking a tranquil forest or a peaceful rainy day, and planting it right in your bedroom, a song woven from the heart of nature.

Brown Noise

Finally, we have brown noise, the mellow baritone. Brown noise, named after the scientist Robert Brown, is deeper and richer, emphasizing the lower frequencies. It is similar to a waterfall's roar or the steady roll of distant thunder, a low-frequency lullaby that hums you into the world of dreams.

With its deep, rhythmic drone, brown noise is incredibly soothing, especially for those who find white noise too static or high-pitched.

Navigating the soundscape of sleep can be a personal journey. It is about discovering the musician—be it white, blue, green, or brown noise—that plays the notes your mind finds most soothing. Each carries its own melody, its own unique promise of peaceful sleep, of nights spent cradled in the soft embrace of restful slumber rather than tossing and turning in frustration.

Understanding these different colors of noise can help you orchestrate your perfect sleep symphony. As you experiment, embrace that sound. Let it fill your room, your nights, your sleep. Rest in its rhythm, let it serenade you into the soothing depths of dreamland, and enjoy the rejuvenation that a night of restful sleep brings.

Next, explore the transformative power of these two sleep remedies designed to create a soothing soundscape, promoting more profound, uninterrupted slumber.

Sleep Remedy One: White Noise Machine

As a sleep enthusiast, I am a big proponent of utilizing noise machines or even handy smartphone apps that emit a spectrum of colored noise, including white, brown, green, or blue. These magical devices are crucial for blanketing environmental sounds that might disrupt sleep. These ambient noises can usher you into a serene slumber by creating a constant and gentle soundscape. Understanding and harnessing their power can make a world of difference to your nighttime routine and overall sleep quality.

Sleep Remedy Two: Lavender Linen Spray

Mix half a cup of purified water, a spoonful of witch hazel, and ten droplets of lavender essential oil in a mist bottle. Agitate thoroughly and gently mist onto your pillowcases, bed sheets, and comforters before retiring for the night. This creates a soothing, aromatic ambiance conducive to rest.

Bonus Remedy: Lavender and Magnesium Relaxing Body Spray

Combine 1/4 cup of magnesium oil and 10 droplets of lavender essential oil in a mister. Mist a modest quantity onto your body, targeting regions such as wrists, neck, and foot soles before retiring to bed. Gently rub into the skin. The blend of dermal magnesium use and soothing lavender fragrance can assist in achieving tranquility and enhancing sleep quality.

The next chapter is dedicated to all the sleeping disorders we experience. Are you ready?

Chapter 5:

Decrypting Sleep Disorders From A–Zzz

Insomnia is an indication, not a chaos. It's like an ache. You're not going to provide a patient ache medicine without figuring out what's reasoning the pain. –Judith Owens

Dive into the world of sleep disorders, exploring their prevalence, impact, and the steps toward recognition, understanding, and effective management.

Common Sleep Disorders and Their Impact

Sleep, as peaceful as it seems, is often marred by a range of disturbances known as sleep disorders. From insomnia to narcolepsy, they can significantly impact our health and well-being. Did you know that there are over 80 recognized sleeping disorders? (MedlinePlus, n.d.).

Allow me to unravel some common ones below.

Circadian Rhythm Disorders

Circadian rhythm disorders are the first stop in our alphabetized journey. Individuals suffering from this disorder might find themselves wide awake at night and struggling to stay alert during the day. The effects are not just limited to sleep deprivation but extend to cognitive impairment, impacting performance in work and everyday activities.

Delayed Sleep Phase Syndrome

Next, we have Delayed Sleep Phase Syndrome (DSPS), a subset of circadian rhythm disorders. Individuals suffering from DSPS usually fall asleep very late and face challenges waking up in time for work, school, or social commitments. This misalignment between their sleep schedule and societal norms can lead to chronic sleep deprivation and associated health issues like depression and cardiovascular diseases.

Insomnia

Insomnia, one of the most widely known sleep disorders, is characterized by persistent difficulty falling or staying asleep. It can wreak havoc on one's daily life, leading to daytime fatigue, poor concentration, mood disturbances, and overall decreased quality of life.

Narcolepsy

When it comes to sleep disorders, narcolepsy stands as a particularly potent condition. Known for excessive daytime sleepiness, sudden loss of muscle control (cataplexy), sleep paralysis, and hallucinations, it can be severely disruptive. Individuals with narcolepsy might find maintaining an active, everyday life challenging due to sudden sleep attacks.

Night Terrors

Night terrors, more common in children, are episodes of screaming, intense fear, and flailing during sleep. They can be terrifying for parents and disruptive to the child's sleep. Although most children outgrow night terrors, the episodes can lead to chronic sleep deprivation if not addressed.

Obstructive Sleep Apnea

Obstructive Sleep Apnea (OSA) is a severe disorder where the individual's breathing continuously stops and starts during sleep due to throat muscles intermittently relaxing and blocking the airway. This results in lower-quality sleep and less oxygen reaching the brain, leading to daytime sleepiness, cognitive dysfunction, and increased risk of heart disease.

Periodic Limb Movement Disorder

Next up, we have Periodic Limb Movement Disorder (PLMD), a condition where a person involuntarily flexes and extends their limbs in sleep. This can lead to disturbed sleep and daytime fatigue, impacting productivity and overall quality of life.

REM Sleep Behavior Disorder

REM Sleep Behavior Disorder (RBD) involves individuals physically acting out vivid dreams, often violent in nature, during REM sleep. It can lead to self-injury or injury to the bed partner, creating a hazardous sleep environment.

Restless Legs Syndrome)

Restless Leg Syndrome (RLS) is known as an irresistible urge to move one's legs and typically occurs during periods of rest or inactivity, especially at night. It can make falling or staying asleep difficult, leading to insomnia and daytime sleepiness.

Sleep Paralysis

Sleep paralysis, the temporary incapacity to speak or move while falling asleep or upon waking, can be a frightening experience. While usually harmless and lasting only a few minutes, it can cause significant distress and disrupt the sleep cycle.

Sleepwalking

Last but certainly not least, we have sleepwalking. This disorder involves complex behaviors like walking, talking, or even driving during deep sleep. Sleepwalking can lead to self-injury and sleep disruption, with consequences that range from simple fatigue to severe physical harm.

Understanding these sleep disorders' impacts and characteristics allows us to better appreciate the intricate dance between sleep and health. Whether you or a loved one are grappling with one of these conditions, knowing what you are facing is the first step toward seeking help and navigating forward to a future of better sleep.

Did You Know?

The average person typically falls asleep within 10–15 minutes of retiring for the night, which reflects a healthy sleep latency. Sleep latency is the time it takes for an individual to transition from full wakefulness to sleep, and this quick transition suggests a good balance between sleep drive and circadian rhythm.

The body's circadian rhythm governs our readiness for sleep. Concurrently, our sleep drive, which builds up the longer we have been awake, creates pressure to sleep. When these two factors align, we feel tired and ready for bed.

If someone falls asleep too quickly, it may indicate excessive sleepiness or potential sleep deprivation. On the other hand, taking too long to fall asleep could signify insomnia or delayed sleep phase disorder.

Achieving that 10–15 minute sleep latency typically means that the individual has good sleep hygiene practices, such as a consistent sleep schedule, a calming presleep routine, and a sleep-conducive environment, thereby aiding the transition into sleep (feather&black, n.d.).

So now that I have unpacked the problems, what exactly are the solutions, you ask?

Techniques for Managing Stress and Treating Sleep Disorders

Max's journey into the labyrinth of sleep and stress was an odyssey neither anticipated nor welcomed. He was a creature of habit, perpetually on the move, juggling the demands of a high-pressure job while trying to maintain a semblance of a personal life. Life was an unrelenting marathon, a race against time he seemed destined to lose. It wasn't until his sleep began to fray at the edges that he understood he was embroiled in a battle he needed to confront head-on.

Max's initial skirmishes with sleeplessness were sporadic, just an off night here or there, dismissed as the byproduct of an overworked mind. However, as the weeks folded into months, those solitary, restless nights amassed into a chronic pattern. His sleep became a maddening enigma, an elusive sprite that darted just beyond reach, leaving him tossing and turning, ensnared in a no-man's-land between consciousness and the realm of dreams.

His daytime vigor waned, and his focus blurred. His mind, once a precision instrument, felt fogged. Tasks that used to be second nature became Herculean challenges. His moods, once steady, became erratic, his patience threadbare. He recognized that his life, work, and relationships were all paying the price.

Max decided it was time to fight back.

His first weapon against this invisible foe was to understand it. After research and consultations, Max was diagnosed with a blend of insomnia and stress-induced circadian rhythm disorder. His high-pressure work environment, coupled with irregular sleep habits, had instigated a dual affliction: his body was stuck in a vicious loop of stress and erratic sleep patterns.

Next, Max decided to court sleep by creating an inviting sleep environment. He replaced his worn-out mattress and his frayed pillows and invested in blackout curtains to shield against intrusive light. He began to treat his bedroom as a sanctuary, reserved solely for sleep and relaxation.

Simultaneously, Max embarked on a mission to regulate his internal clock. He set strict sleep and wake times and adhered to a calming prebedtime routine that included journaling and blowing bubbles. He experimented with different colored noises, finding that the soothing hum of brown noise, akin to a distant waterfall, lulled him into a gentle slumber.

For stress, Max turned to mindfulness techniques, including volunteering at his local animal shelter and swimming. He attended cognitive behavioral therapy sessions where he learned to manage his stress and reframe his thinking. He even picked up fluid intuitive dance, the flowy movements becoming a trance of relaxation, a physical meditation that drained away the tension coiled within him.

Max's nutritional choices also saw a sea change. He focused on a balanced diet, limited caffeine, and avoided heavy meals close to bedtime. He embraced regular physical activity, understanding how exercise helped manage his stress levels and promoted better sleep.

His journey was not linear, his progress not always immediate, but Max remained undeterred. There were nights he lay awake, frustration gnawing at him. But he would remind himself, as his therapist taught him, that a poor night of sleep was not a failure but part of the process.

Slowly, Max began to reclaim his nights. His sleepless episodes dwindled, and his stress levels began to abate. He felt rejuvenated, the fog lifted, and his moods stabilized. His work flourished, and his personal life thrived. The marathon of life still raged on, but now, he was no longer running on empty. His sleep had become his ally, his stress a foe he had learned to tame.

Max's journey through the sleep-stress nexus was not easy, nor was it swift. But his odyssey led to an understanding, an appreciation of his body's needs and the importance of balance. He recognized that his sleep was not just an off switch at the end of the day but a vital, powerful tool that could either fuel or hinder his life.

Sleep disorders and stress can be formidable adversaries, but as Max discovered, they are not insurmountable. By understanding the nuances of his body, embracing positive lifestyle changes, and seeking professional help, Max navigated his way to healthier sleep and a less stressful life. His journey is a testament to the resilience and the power of understanding one's own body and mind.

Explore the transformative sleep methods below, designed to enhance your slumber, rejuvenate your body, and optimize your overall well-being.

Sleep Remedy One: Relaxation Exercises for Insomnia

Embrace techniques like progressive muscle relaxation, visually guided journeys, or aromatherapy to soothe your body and pacify your mind, offering relief from insomnia.

Method 1: Progressive Muscle Relaxation

Intentionally strain and relax your various muscle groups, facilitating a sense of calm and dissipating bodily tension. This practice helps release stress-related physical discomfort, fostering an environment conducive to sleep.

Method 2: Guided Imagery

Visualize yourself in serene, comforting surroundings, harnessing your senses to foster a relaxing and soothing state. This method engages your mind in positive imagery, easing anxious thoughts and promoting mental relaxation for better sleep.

Method 3: Aromatherapy

Aromatherapy uses essential oils like lavender and chamomile to stimulate brain functions, reducing anxiety and promoting relaxation, thereby improving sleep quality. Inhaling these scents triggers a calming response in the brain, enhancing your overall sleep environment.

Sleep Remedy Two: Sleep-Inducing Herbal Tea

Allow a medley of valerian root, passionflower, and lemon balm to infuse in boiling water for a span of 10 minutes. Recognized for their tranquilizing attributes, these herbs aid in fostering a relaxed state prior to slumber. Consuming the tea roughly 30 minutes before retiring can yield the best outcomes. Make tea time your new sleepy time routine!

Did You Know?

While it is not entirely clear why some people sleepwalk, an estimated 15% of the American population does so, often leading to complex, sometimes dangerous behaviors during sleep. Sleepwalking, or somnambulism, typically occurs during deep sleep and can result in actions as simple as sitting up in bed or as elaborate as leaving the house and driving a car.

The exact cause of sleepwalking is not known, but it appears to run in families, indicating a potential genetic link. In addition, sleep deprivation, irregular sleep schedules, and certain medications can trigger episodes. Stress and alcohol consumption can also play a role.

Interestingly, sleepwalking is more common in children, especially those between the ages of three and seven. However, most children outgrow sleepwalking by their teen years. In adults, sleepwalking is often linked to other sleep disorders, such as sleep apnea or RLS.

Despite its prevalence, sleepwalking is usually not a cause for concern unless it leads to harmful behaviors or interferes with restful sleep. If it does, professional medical advice should be sought to manage and mitigate the condition's effects (feather&black, n.d.).

Next, I will unveil the power of magnesium in our sleeping patterns.

Chapter 6:

Magnesium's Role in Stress and Sleep

Magnesium oil has the ability to increase the body's production of DHEA, a hormone that has beneficial effects on memory, stress, sleep, and depression… –Carolyn Dean

Magnesium, an essential mineral, is pivotal in managing stress and promoting restful sleep. Discover its influence on our nervous system, circadian rhythm, and overall well-being as we delve into the intriguing connection between magnesium, stress, and sleep.

How Anxiety, Stress, and Sleep Quality Are Intertwined

Understanding the intricate dance between stress, anxiety, and sleep can seem like unraveling a tightly knotted ball of twine. However, it is a connection worth dissecting, given its profound impact on our wellness. This complex relationship is often bidirectional, meaning that stress can precipitate disrupted sleep, and inversely, inadequate sleep can heighten stress and anxiety levels.

Consider a seminal study conducted by Harvard Medical School. It elucidated how stress instigates a hormonal cascade spearheaded by cortisol—the quintessential stress hormone.

Cortisol, typically higher during the day, dwindles toward nighttime, preparing our bodies for sleep. But when stress strikes, cortisol remains elevated, thus disrupting our circadian rhythm and impeding the initiation of sleep (Harvard Health Publishing, 2020).

It is not just sleep initiation that is affected. A few years ago, a published study suggested that heightened stress might precipitate fragmented sleep, increased REM sleep, and reduced deep, restorative non-REM sleep. This broken, shallow sleep fails to fully restore us, leaving us feeling weary and sluggish (Kim & Dimsdale, 2007).

Now, let me turn the lens around. How does poor sleep contribute to escalating stress and anxiety levels? Here, we turn to sleep debt or cumulative lack of sleep. A recent study established a direct correlation between sleep debt and heightened cortisol levels. When we are deprived of sleep, our cortisol levels surge, instigating feelings of stress and anxiety and fostering a vicious cycle (Hackett et al., 2020).

Chronic stress and anxiety carve a deeper, more insidious impact on our sleep and overall health. According to a publication from 2020, persistent high stress and anxiety can lead to insomnia and other sleep disorders. The ramifications extend beyond the night. Poor sleep affects our cognitive functions, mental health, cardiovascular health, and even our metabolic health, creating a ripple effect on our overall well-being (Kaur et al., 2020).

That is the intricate tapestry woven by stress, anxiety, and sleep—a tapestry that can seem overwhelmingly tangled. Recognizing this interplay is the first step toward untangling it. By acknowledging the impact of stress on our sleep and vice versa, we can adopt targeted strategies to manage stress and improve sleep, thereby breaking the cycle. It is not always easy, but given the profound health implications, it is a journey worth embarking upon.

Many scientific studies suggest the benefits of stress management techniques like cognitive behavioral therapy, mindfulness, and other relaxing prebed activities in promoting better sleep. Simultaneously, improving sleep hygiene—maintaining regular sleep-wake schedules, curating a conducive sleep environment, and avoiding sleep disruptors like caffeine and electronic devices before bed—can help manage stress and anxiety.

Did You Know?

Sleep plays a crucial role in our immune system's functionality. During sleep, particularly during the deep stages of sleep, the body produces and releases various immune cells like cytokines, T cells, and interleukin 12. Cytokines are proteins that regulate the body's response to infection and inflammation. Some cytokines also help promote sleep, meaning getting enough sleep can enhance their production.

In addition, infection-fighting cells and antibodies are decreased when you do not get enough sleep, making the body more susceptible to illnesses. For instance, studies have shown that people who don't get enough sleep are likelier to get sick after exposure to a virus, such as a common cold. Sleep deprivation can also impact how fast you recover if you get sick.

On the other hand, sufficient sleep can boost the effectiveness of specific specialized immune cells called T cells. Unlike other immune cells, T cells fight against intracellular pathogens, for example, virus-infected cells such as flu, HIV, herpes, and cancer cells. During sleep, these T cells can adhere better to their targets and hence are more efficient in their function. Therefore, getting adequate sleep promotes the immune system's optimal functioning and helps us stay healthy (feather&black, n.d.).

Let us now look at the soothing impact of magnesium.

The Calming Effects of Magnesium on the Nervous System

Magnesium: Did you know it is the fourth most plentiful mineral in your body? It is needed for over 300 biochemical reactions (Office of Dietary Supplements, 2022).

It is the unsung hero in our wellness narrative, influencing everything from nerve function to muscle relaxation to the regulation of stress hormones. Yet, its role in stress management and sleep enhancement is often underplayed.

Let me begin by helping you understand magnesium's role in our bodies. It is a critical cog in the functioning of our nervous system. According to a review, magnesium modulates synaptic density and plasticity, which, in effect, means it helps neurons "communicate" better. It is also the watchman of the N-methyl-D-aspartate (NMDA) receptor, a gateway for calcium ions, which, when unchecked, can overexcite neurons and lead to neurodegeneration (Jewett & Thapa, 2020).

Secondly, magnesium is our muscle's best friend. A study published in the 80s detailed how magnesium aids muscle relaxation by countering calcium, which induces muscle contraction. This magnesium-calcium interplay is integral in maintaining healthy muscle function (Potter et al., 1981).

Thirdly, let us explore magnesium's influence on our stress response. It is an adrenal gland regulator—the key to our body's stress response. A paper published a few years ago posited that low magnesium levels can upregulate the production of stress hormones like cortisol (Pickering et al., 2020).

Now that we have grasped magnesium's vital roles, let us delve into its potential benefits for stress reduction and improved sleep quality. A review some years back presented compelling evidence for magnesium supplementation as a natural remedy for anxiety. It is hypothesized that by improving synaptic function, reducing neuronal excitability, and dampening the stress response, magnesium might exert anxiolytic effects (Boyle et al., 2017).

Similarly, several studies have hinted at a possible connection between magnesium and sleep quality. A publication concluded that dietary magnesium supplementation could increase subjective insomnia measures, such as sleep efficiency and sleep time (Abbasi et al., 2012).

But where can we find this remarkable mineral? Magnesium-rich food sources are plentiful and diverse. Leafy greens like spinach, whole grains, nuts, seeds, and dark chocolate are treasure troves of magnesium. Even tap and bottled water can contribute to our magnesium intake (Spirtzler, 2018).

However, the key is not just consuming magnesium but maintaining adequate levels. A survey warned that less than 60% of the American adult population achieved the recommended dietary allowance for magnesium. Such deficiencies can impair our nervous system function, muscle relaxation, and stress response and potentially rob us of the additional benefits magnesium might offer in terms of anxiety reduction and sleep improvement (World Health Organization, 2005).

In conclusion, magnesium's multifaceted roles in our bodies underscore its importance in our wellness journey. By appreciating its functions and potential benefits, we can make more informed dietary choices, maintain adequate magnesium levels, and possibly enjoy a more serene mind and restful sleep.

Finally, let's discover two sleep methods to rejuvenate your nights, replenish your energy, and profoundly transform your waking life. Does breakfast for dinner sound good? Great!

Sleep Remedy One: Cocoa and Almond Butter Smoothie

Blend 1 tablespoon cocoa powder, 1 tablespoon almond butter, 1 cup almond milk, 1/2 banana, and ice cubes. Savor before sleep. Cocoa's tryptophan and almond butter's magnesium promote relaxation and potential melatonin synthesis.

Sleep Remedy Two: Cinnamon Banana Overnight Oats

In a jar, combine 1/2 cup rolled oats, 1/2 mashed banana, 1/2 cup milk (dairy or plant-based), 1/2 teaspoon cinnamon, and a drizzle of honey. Stir, cover, and refrigerate overnight. Enjoy as a comforting dinner option and prepare for sleepy time! Oats offer serotonin-boosting vitamin B6, while bananas provide natural sugars. Cinnamon's warmth adds a soothing touch for bedtime.

Next, we will explore how technology can be used for good or evil when it comes to sleep.

Chapter 7:

The Battle Between Tech and Sleep

"Go to sleep, you'll feel better tomorrow" is the human version of "Did you try turning it off and on again?" –BedBreeZzz Media

Delve into how nighttime technology use can hijack our sleep, disrupting our rest and unraveling our body's natural rhythm. Let me illuminate the shadows.

The Effects of Tech on Sleep Quality

Did you know modern technology impacts your slumber, alters sleep quality, and potentially reshapes your entire well-being? Let me explain below.

Blue Light and Disruptive Sleep Patterns

Have you ever wondered why, despite your physical exhaustion, sleep sometimes seems to play hard to get after a long day of screen time? Let me dive into the mystery of blue light emission, a ubiquitous aspect of our digital lives, and its impacts on our sleep quality.

Our journey starts within the human eye with a light-sensitive protein called melanopsin. Discovered relatively recently, in

2002, melanopsin is found in special cells in the retina known as intrinsically photosensitive retinal ganglion cells. When these cells detect blue light wavelengths, usually abundant in morning sunlight, they signal the brain's master clock—the SCN—that it is time to be awake (Lazzerini Ospri et al., 2017).

In response, the SCN orchestrates the release of cortisol, a hormone that helps us feel alert while suppressing melatonin. In essence, blue light acts as a wakefulness trigger in the context of our natural circadian rhythm.

However, the advent of artificial lighting and electronic devices has changed our relationship with light and darkness. Modern screens, from smartphones to tablets to laptops, emit substantial amounts of blue light, and if we use these devices in the evening, our retinas may perceive it as morning, sending confusing signals to our SCN.

Multiple studies reflect the impacts of evening blue light exposure. A recent report showed that exposure to blue-enriched light in the evening significantly suppressed melatonin production and delayed the timing of our internal clock (Wahl et al., 2019).

Another study further illuminated the link between nighttime screen use and sleep issues. Participants who used screens more in the hours before sleep reported increased difficulty falling asleep and decreased sleep quality. The researcher concluded that high exposure to screen light before bed is a risk factor for sleep disturbances (Hale, 2018).

The impact is not only on sleep duration and quality. Sleep timing, often overlooked, is equally crucial. Researchers found that blue light shifts the circadian rhythm twice as much as green light, potentially pushing our sleep-wake cycle out of alignment with our social and work schedules (Wahl et al., 2019).

What, then, can we do about our digital lives? Solutions range from software fixes like "night mode" on devices, which reduces blue light emission, to wearing blue-light-blocking glasses in the evening. However, perhaps the most effective remedy is maintaining good "light hygiene"— maximizing natural light exposure in the morning, reducing artificial light in the evening, and turning off screens at least an hour before bed.

In conclusion, the tale of blue light is a poignant reminder of the subtle ways our modern lifestyle can interfere with ancient biological rhythms. By understanding how blue light affects our sleep, we can be more mindful of our screen time, especially in the hours leading up to bedtime.

Late Night Screen Time and Melatonin Production

Consider this scenario: It is late at night, and you are nestled comfortably in bed, but instead of drifting off to sleep, you are engrossed in a fascinating article on your smartphone. Seems harmless, right? But this routine, shared by many of us in the digital age, has a surprising impact on our sleep biology, particularly on the hormone that ushers us into dreamland: melatonin.

As we have already discussed, melatonin is a critical player in our body's sleep-wake cycle, also known as the circadian rhythm. Under normal conditions, melatonin levels rise in the late evening, remain high throughout the night, and drop in the early morning. This rise and fall in melatonin promotes sleep and helps set the timing of our internal biological clock.

Enter the ubiquitous screen—be it a smartphone, tablet, computer, or TV. These devices emit substantial amounts of light at the blue end of the spectrum. While all light can suppress melatonin production to some extent, blue light, owing to its shorter wavelength, does so more powerfully.

We have also recently discovered that when we expose ourselves to screen light in the evening, the blue light detected by the eyes sends a signal to the brain's SCN. The SCN responds as if it were daylight, suppressing melatonin production and delaying sleep onset.

Several scientific studies have lent weight to this. Research conducted a few years back found that individuals who read from a light-emitting e-reader before bedtime took longer to fall asleep, had reduced evening sleepiness, and decreased melatonin secretion compared to those reading a printed book (Chang et al., 2014).

Another published study analyzed data from over 20,000 participants and concluded that bedtime screen use was associated with insufficient sleep duration, poor sleep quality, and excessive daytime sleepiness (AlShareef, 2022).

These findings are particularly concerning given screens' widespread evening use and melatonin's important role in facilitating sleep. Disruptions to melatonin rhythms have been linked to insomnia, poor sleep quality, and various health issues, including mood disorders, metabolic syndrome, and even certain types of cancer.

So, what can be done to mitigate these effects? One immediate solution is to minimize screen usage in the hours leading up to bedtime. The National Sleep Foundation advises putting down all electronic devices at least 60 minutes before bed to allow melatonin levels to rise normally.

If you absolutely need to use a device in the evening, consider adjusting your screen settings. Many modern devices now offer a "night shift" or similar feature that reduces the amount of blue light emitted. Alternatively, blue light-blocking glasses can also be used to filter out the blue light.

A final and perhaps more holistic solution is cultivating a mindful relationship with our devices. By becoming aware of our screen habits and their impact on our sleep, we can make healthier choices—like reading a physical book or practicing relaxation before bed, rather than reaching for the phone.

While screens have become a non-negotiable part of modern life, their impact on sleep is a genuine concern. By understanding the mechanisms, namely the suppression of melatonin production, we can make informed choices about our screen use, protect our sleep, and thus, safeguard our health.

Now that we have defined the problem, let us explore some solutions together using stories from real people.

Did You Know?

Fascinatingly, sleep patterns often vary between men and women, influenced by biological, hormonal, and lifestyle differences. Women, in general, require slightly more sleep than men, about 20 minutes more on average, according to sleep researchers. This difference is believed to be due to women's multitasking brains that expend more energy during the day, necessitating more recovery time during sleep. Furthermore, the menstrual cycle, pregnancy, and menopause introduce hormonal changes that can significantly affect sleep patterns and quality in women. For example, fluctuations in progesterone and estrogen can lead to insomnia or disturbed sleep. On the other hand, men have a higher prevalence of sleep apnea, a disorder that interrupts breathing during sleep, often leading to fragmented and less restful sleep. These differences emphasize the importance of individualized sleep health strategies (feather&black, n.d.).

Strategies for Reducing Tech Before Sleep

Dive into practical strategies to lessen tech usage before bed, fostering healthier habits for a restful, rejuvenating night's sleep in our tech-driven world.

The Digital Curfew

Angela was a vibrant soul who thrived in the digital world, relishing every byte of information that flowed through her fingertips. Her phone was a constant companion, like an extension of herself, until she realized that this digital tether was robbing her of something precious: sleep. Nights that should have been dedicated to restful slumber became battlegrounds, with Angela wrestling with a barrage of emails, social media updates, and captivating videos. The bleary-eyed mornings and caffeine-fueled days were a harsh price to pay for the stolen hours of sleep.

Recognizing the havoc her habits were wreaking on her well-being, Angela knew it was time for a change. She stumbled upon the concept of a digital curfew—a self-imposed restriction on using electronic devices after a particular hour. Intrigued, she committed to turning off her devices an hour before bedtime, despite the initial challenge of disconnecting from her digital life.

The first few nights were tough, with Angela fidgeting restlessly, her mind seemingly in a state of withdrawal. She reached for her phone, only to remember the silent promise she had made to herself. The siren call of notifications was challenging to resist, yet with every passing day, the urge diminished a bit more.

Slowly but surely, Angela started seeing a change. Her mind felt less cluttered in the quiet hours before sleep, and she fell asleep faster, her dreams no longer invaded by phantom rings or imagined updates. With the brain fog lifting, her mornings became more pleasant, replaced by a renewed sense of clarity and focus.

Surprisingly, Angela found new appreciation in the offline world during her curfew hours. She started reading physical books, a passion she had neglected in her predigital life. She rekindled her love for drawing, the soothing strokes of the pencil on paper serving as a calming prelude to sleep.

Reflecting on her journey, Angela marveled at the power of the digital curfew. What started as an experiment had transformed into a cherished ritual, a sanctuary from the ceaseless hum of the digital world. Not only did it give her back her sleep, but it also gifted her time—uninterrupted, peaceful moments that were indeed her own.

The tale of Angela's digital curfew inspires all who feel entrapped in the digital web, struggling to find balance. Implementing a digital curfew is not about rejecting technology; it is about drawing a line and creating boundaries that ensure our digital lives do not infringe on our natural sleep cycles. It is about rediscovering the value of disconnected moments, finding tranquility in the silence, and, most importantly, safeguarding our sleep. After all, a well-rested mind is the greatest asset in our hyperconnected world.

The Tech-Free Bedtime Routine

George had always been a night owl, thriving under the moonlight where his creativity soared. His days were consumed by the demands of the bustling tech industry, while the soft glow of screens lit up his nights. Online shopping, reading articles, and endless digital tasks bled into the late hours, blurring the line between daytime and nighttime. His nights became an extension of his waking hours, driving sleep away.

The turning point arrived when George woke up one morning, his body feeling heavy, his mind foggy. He gazed at his reflection and barely recognized the weary eyes staring back at him. He realized he had ignored the toll his habits had taken on his well-being. It was time for a change.

To reclaim his sleep, George decided to take a drastic step—a tech-free bedtime routine. He resolved to banish screens from his bedroom, a decision that felt almost alien in his digitally dominated existence. He created a nightly ritual, a routine devoid of any electronic devices, designed to ease his mind into the kingdom of sleep.

His new routine began with a warm cup of chamomile tea, an age-old remedy known for its calming properties. Next, he spent some time jotting down his thoughts, a brain dump of sorts, releasing the day's chaos onto paper. This was followed by some light reading, losing himself in stories far removed from his digital life.

The first few nights were challenging, the habitual itch to check his phone persisting. His mind craved the stimulation of screens, the constant influx of information. But with each passing night, the longing receded. The rhythm of his routine started to replace the digital cravings, the calming rituals signaling his mind that it was time to sleep.

Before long, George noticed a remarkable change. His sleep was deeper, his mornings brighter. The fog lifted, replaced by a sharpness he had nearly forgotten. His days became more productive, his energy levels soaring. His creative thoughts found a new direction, uncluttered by the noise of the digital world.

The creation of a tech-free bedtime routine transformed George's life. His nights, once held hostage by the digital hemisphere, now belonged to him again. His sleep became a sanctuary, a respite from the world that allowed him to recharge and rejuvenate.

George's story highlights the power of disconnecting. Creating a tech-free bedtime routine does not mean denying the value of technology. It is about crafting a peaceful segue from our busy days to restful nights. It is about honoring the human need for rest and nurturing our minds through restful sleep in a world that never sleeps. It is about reclaiming our nights, one tech-free routine at a time.

Limiting Blue Light Emission From Devices

In the heart of the city that never sleeps lived Jenny, a vibrant artist, her world as colorful as her creations. Her days were filled with hues and textures, but her nights bore the monotonous blue tint of her digital devices. Art was her calling, but technology was her vice, an essential tool in sharing her work with the world. Sleep became an elusive entity with every night spent in the blue glow of her devices.

Jenny's fight with insomnia started as an occasional inconvenience but swiftly morphed into a nightly battle. Tossing and turning became her routine as the melodic rhythm of sleep danced just beyond her grasp. Mornings found her listless and weary; the day ahead seemed like an uphill task.

The insomnia was taking a toll on her creativity. Her colors were losing their vibrancy, her strokes their confidence. This sleep-deprived existence was not the life Jenny wanted to live. She needed a solution.

Upon learning the effects of blue light emission on sleep, Jenny discovered the missing piece of her sleep puzzle. Devices she was glued to late into the night were major culprits, their blue light tricking her brain into believing it was still daytime. The discovery marked the beginning of her sleep transformation journey.

Jenny turned to technology, not to feed her insomnia but to starve it. She discovered apps and features that limited blue light emission on devices. The warmer hues these tools offered were a soothing replacement for the harsh blue light. She set these apps to activate automatically in the evening, reassuring her that the day was winding down and that it was time to prepare for sleep.

At first, the change was strange. The blue that had become so familiar was now replaced with tones of amber. But with each passing night, Jenny began to welcome this change. Her nights no longer felt like an extension of the day but a realm distinct and calming. The evening transition to warmer screen tones began to signal her mind to start its own evolution into rest mode.

Jenny's adoption of these simple digital tools significantly impacted her sleep quality. She began to fall asleep faster, her nights no longer an arena for the battle of insomnia. Her mornings were refreshing, starkly contrasting with the weary dawns she was used to. With restful sleep, her creativity found a new lease on life. Her art flourished, a reflection of her renewed spirit.

Jenny's tale underscores an essential lesson: Technology, often seen as a sleep adversary, can be repurposed into an ally. By embracing tools that limit blue light emission (such as adding screen filters to mobile phones and operating a phone on night mode), we can transform our sleep environment, shielding our nights from the sleep-disrupting effects of our devices. In the quest for better sleep, these small changes can paint a big picture, much like the subtle strokes in Jenny's vibrant masterpieces.

Welcome to two revolutionary sleep methods, described below, promising to transform your nights, promote restful slumber, and rejuvenate your mornings. Discover the magic of sound sleep.

Sleep Remedy One: Blue-Light-Filtering Glasses

Adorn your eyes with blue-light-blocking spectacles in the evening, preventing the sleep-disruptive blue light from your devices. This supports natural melatonin levels, enhancing sleep wellness.

Bonus Remedy: Activate Blue Light Filter on Your Phone

Utilize the built-in blue light filter or "night mode" on your phone in the evening. Adjust the settings to reduce the amount of blue light emitted from your screen. Enabling the blue light filter can help minimize blue light exposure, making it easier for your body to produce melatonin and prepare for sleep.

Sleep Remedy Two: Sleep-Inducing Banana Pancakes

Well, it seems we are back to breakfast for dinner recipes for some delicious reason. In this dish, crush a mature banana to a pulp. Incorporate half a cup of oats, a quarter cup of almond flour, a spoonful of honey, and a dash of cinnamon. Stir thoroughly until it reaches a dough-like texture. Warm a non-stick skillet on medium heat and ladle modest dollops of the mixture onto the hot surface to form petite pancakes. Allow them to brown on each side. Relish this warm, sleep-enhancing delight prior to slumber. Bananas' tryptophan and potassium promote relaxation and sustained sleep.

Next, we will explore the impact of creating a healthy hygiene habit before hitting the sack.

Chapter 8:

Establishing a Nighttime Routine for Sleep Hygiene

Think in the morning. Act in the noon. Eat in the evening. Sleep in the night. –William Blake

Embark on a journey to impeccable sleep hygiene as we establish a nighttime routine that encourages restful, rejuvenating sleep.

Promoting Restful Sleep Through Healthy Sleep Hygiene Habits

Unearth the secret to restful slumber as we explore how healthy sleep hygiene habits foster deeper, more satisfying sleep and invigorated mornings.

The Significance of Consistent Sleep Schedules and Regular Sleep-Wake Times

Harnessing the power of consistent sleep schedules and regular sleep-wake times is vital in pursuing optimal sleep quality and overall well-being. Our bodies thrive on regularity, thanks to our circadian rhythm. This clock dictates when we feel alert and when we feel tired.

The rhythm is ingrained in us. However, we can disrupt it with erratic sleep patterns. Going to bed and waking up at the same time daily reinforces this rhythm, helping us fall asleep quicker and have more restful sleep. When we deviate from our schedule—sleeping in on weekends, for example—we may experience the equivalent of jet lag, known as "social jet lag."

Having a regular sleep-wake schedule also helps regulate our sleep stages, specifically deep sleep and REM sleep. Deep sleep, the most restorative sleep stage, primarily occurs in the first half of the night. REM sleep, during which we dream, happens predominantly in the second half. Irregular sleep schedules can interrupt these stages, leading to poor sleep quality.

But maintaining a consistent sleep schedule goes beyond simply deciding when to turn in and when to rise. It is also about building an evening routine that cues your body's bedtime. This could involve activities such as threading beads, receiving a gentle massage, or building a puzzle, done consistently and sequentially, leading up to bedtime.

While setting a regular sleep-wake schedule, it is essential to be realistic about your sleep needs and lifestyle. Consider when you naturally feel tired and when you need to wake up for work or school. From there, work backward to determine an ideal bedtime.

Even with a consistent sleep schedule, we might sometimes have trouble falling asleep. If you find yourself tossing and turning after 20 minutes, it is best to get out of bed and do a quiet activity in dim light until you feel sleepy. Lying awake can create an unhealthy link between your mattress and wakefulness.

In conclusion, when complemented with other good sleep hygiene practices, a regular sleep-wake schedule can significantly enhance sleep quality. A consistent program improves sleep and has broad implications for physical and mental health, enhancing alertness, mood, and cognitive function. Regular sleep schedules are one of the most powerful yet underutilized tools to improve sleep, health, and quality of life.

The Impact of a Relaxing Bedtime Routine on Sleep Quality

Imagine your mind as a bustling city at peak hour and sleep as the quiet countryside. A relaxing bedtime routine is the bridge that gently and predictably carries you from your day's noise to the night's tranquility.

Cultivating a comfortable presleep routine is a powerful tool in your sleep hygiene arsenal. It is not merely about what we do in the hour or two before bed but how these activities help transition our body and mind from wakefulness to sleep. They signal our brain that it is time to wind down, helping regulate our circadian rhythm and encouraging melatonin's timely release.

Let me delve into some components of an effective bedtime routine and their influence on sleep quality.

Firstly, consider the environment. Create a sleep-friendly atmosphere in your bedroom. This means a cool, dark, and quiet room, preferably with no distractions like a TV or work materials. Some find the addition of calming elements like lavender scent or white noise helpful.

Incorporate relaxation techniques. Practices such as gratitude exercises, deep breathing exercises, progressive muscle relaxation, or static stretches can effectively reduce heart rate, blood pressure, and stress hormones, preparing your body for sleep.

Engage in calming activities. Writing down your to-do list for tomorrow, listening to gentle music, or maintaining a comfortable room temperature are all examples. These activities should be enjoyable, easy to do, and free from stress triggers.

Adopt a consistent sleep program. Sleeping and waking up at the same time every day, even on weekends, promotes your internal clock, making it more straightforward to fall asleep and wake up.

Lastly, establish a presleep ritual that suits you. Everyone's preferences and needs are different. What works for one person may not work for another. Your bedtime routine should be something you look forward to, not a chore.

The benefits of a relaxing bedtime routine extend beyond improved sleep quality. Better sleep contributes to enhanced mood, higher energy levels, improved cognitive function, and overall better health. Furthermore, the routine provides a structured end to the day, offering a mental respite from the stress and demands of daily life.

However, remember that change takes time. Implementing a new routine requires patience and consistency. The effects may not be immediate, but persistence pays off.

To summarize, a relaxing bedtime routine is a practical and holistic approach to improving sleep quality. It acts as a gentle nudge, telling our body and mind, "It's time for sleep." Each person's journey to better sleep is unique, so explore, experiment, and find what works best for you.

Did You Know?

An intriguing fact is that humans, unlike many other mammals, can't willingly delay sleep for extended periods without experiencing adverse health and cognitive impacts. This is primarily due to our circadian rhythms, which are roughly 24-hour cycles influencing our sleep-wake patterns. While some animals can adjust their sleep cycles based on needs like hunting or avoiding predators, humans' sleep-wake cycles are less flexible. Prolonged sleep deprivation in humans leads to significant cognitive impairments and mood disruptions and can increase the chances of medical conditions like heart disease and diabetes (feather&black, n.d.).

Strategies for Creating a Constant Bedtime Routine

The moon painted the world silver as Lily, a freelance graphic designer, clocked out from her home office. She found herself facing a common but taxing issue: irregular sleep patterns. Nighttime had become a roulette wheel of possibilities—insomnia, fitful slumber, or unexpected awakenings. She yearned for a peaceful night's sleep but struggled to understand how to achieve it.

A friend suggested a constant bedtime routine, explaining that this strategy could provide the structure her sleep cycle needed. Intrigued and hopeful, Lily decided to construct her unique presleep ritual.

The first strategy Lily tried was the simple act of dimming the lights around her home as nighttime descended. This adjustment was minor but had profound effects. Lowered lighting signaled her brain that day was turning into night, mirroring the environmental cues our ancestors followed. This small change created a gentle, environmental whisper that nudged her toward drowsiness, a nudge she found surprisingly effective.

Lily incorporated a warm bath into her routine to enhance her sleep environment, usually around an hour before her decided bedtime. The gentle heat relaxed her muscles, physically washing away the tension from her work. As she stepped out of the bath, the cooler air of her bedroom promoted a drop in body temperature, which induced a sleepy sensation.

Being a creative individual, she also discovered a love for aromatherapy. Lily found lavender oil, a scent long associated with relaxation, her favorite. A few drops in her bathwater, and the smell would linger on her skin, following her to bed, providing a soft, aromatic lullaby.

While setting up these positive habits, Lily recognized the importance of steering clear of certain activities before bedtime. One such stimulant was her love for evening workouts. She realized her adrenaline-pumping, heart-racing exercise routine kept her alert far into the night. She moved her workouts to mornings, replacing them with gentle stretches and deep-breathing exercises in the evening. This helped her wind down physically and mentally, releasing stress and preparing her body for sleep.

She also started monitoring her caffeine intake. She had a habit of drinking tea well into the evening. Switching her evening cup to a decaffeinated herbal blend, she noticed a difference. The reduction in caffeine allowed her body to recognize and respond to its natural sleep cues.

At first, the process was slow. Change always is. But Lily did not let the initial struggle discourage her. She remained consistent, understanding that her body needed time to adapt to these changes. After a few weeks, Lily began noticing improvements. Falling asleep became easier. The sleep she got was deeper and more restful. She woke up feeling rejuvenated and ready for the day.

Lily learned that a consistent bedtime routine, tailored to her preferences and lifestyle, wasn't just about promoting better sleep. It also provided her with a structured period of relaxation and self-care. It was her time—a soothing end to her day, a gentle bridge to a restful night.

In her journey, Lily discovered that crafting a constant bedtime routine isn't a one-size-fits-all solution. It is personal and flexible. It's about finding what works for you and what doesn't. It is about being kind to yourself and understanding that your path to better sleep is unique.

Through the dimming of lights, the warmth of a bath, the comfort of a chosen aroma, and by avoiding late-night stimulants, Lily constructed her bedtime routine. It was a personal blend of strategies uniquely designed for her. And it worked. For Lily, the path to a good night's sleep was no longer a chaotic scramble in the dark but a gentle, predictable stroll under the moonlight.

Depart on a deeper sleep journey with the remedies below if you still find yourself struggling at night.

Sleep Remedy One: Journaling for Better Sleep

Maintain a diary nearby while you prepare to sleep, and take a moment to pen down daily contemplations, anxieties, or musings. It aids in mental detoxification and encourages tranquility.

Sleep Remedy Two: Banana and Peanut Butter Toast

Spread peanut butter on whole-grain toast and top with banana slices. Enjoy as a light evening snack. Bananas' tryptophan and peanuts' magnesium support relaxation and neurotransmitter production.

Do you know that feeling when taking a glorious afternoon nap? Next up, we will unveil the power of a nap. Stay tuned!

Chapter 9:

The Power of Napping for Enhanced Productivity

A day without a nap is like a cupcake without frosting. –Terri Guillemets

Unleash untapped energy and boost productivity with the revitalizing power of strategic napping, a potent tool in your personal wellness toolkit. Explore its magic within.

The Benefits of Napping for Energy and Cognitive Function

Did you know? NASA found naps can increase alertness by 100% (Meyer, 2014). Explore how napping refuels energy and sharpens cognition in this invigorating chapter.

The Concept of Power Naps

Ever felt that midday slump where your energy levels drop, and concentration seems impossible? This is where the concept of a "power nap" steps in. It is not your typical leisurely afternoon siesta but a short, quick, and efficient burst of rest that replenishes your energy reserves, leaving you refreshed and alert.

Despite their brevity—usually 10 to 30 minutes—power naps are potent against fatigue, transforming your day by providing an instant energy surge. The secret lies in limiting the nap's duration, thus preventing entry into deep sleep stages, which results in sleep inertia or grogginess upon waking.

Numerous scientific studies extol the benefits of power napping. A study showed that a 20-minute nap significantly enhances cognitive functioning and alertness (Lovato & Lack, 2010). Meanwhile, other research demonstrated that a short nap could substantially improve learning and memory (Cousins et al., 2018).

Power napping is not just about closing your eyes for a few minutes; it's a process that requires a proper setting and time management. Choosing a quiet, dimly lit room can aid in quickly falling asleep, while setting an alarm ensures you do not oversleep and disrupt your nighttime sleep.

It is also crucial to understand the best time for power napping. It has been suggested that early to mid-afternoon, around 2–3 p.m., is ideal. This timing aligns with your body's natural circadian rhythm, when most people experience a post-lunch dip in energy (Summer, 2020).

Moreover, power naps can benefit those with sleep deficits. A power nap can help alleviate sleep deprivation by supplementing lost nighttime sleep, leading to improved mood, reduced stress, better reaction time, and increased patience.

Despite its benefits, power napping is not for everyone. For instance, individuals with insomnia or difficulty sleeping at night may find that napping exacerbates their problems. Additionally, those who experience sleep inertia, a feeling of grogginess and disorientation after waking, may find power naps more detrimental than beneficial.

Power napping is a skill, much like meditation, that can be cultivated with practice. The goal is to awaken just before deep sleep begins. With time, many individuals can master this delicate balance, deriving maximum energy and alertness benefits from their daytime slumbers.

Power napping, a simple yet effective tool, promises an energy revival that coffee cannot match—and without the unpleasant side effects. Understanding and harnessing the power of this brief rest can enhance productivity, invigorate your mind, and bring balance to your busy day.

How Short Naps Improve Alertness, Attention, and Productivity

Boosting Alertness

Imagine a scenario where your eyelids are heavy, your focus falters, and you yearn for an instant burst of alertness. That is precisely where short naps step in, rejuvenating your senses and enhancing your alertness.

A brief nap stimulates specific brain activities, improving alertness and promoting wakefulness. The key lies in timing your rest perfectly, ensuring it is short enough to avoid slipping into a deep sleep, which may leave you groggy and disoriented. By recharging your mental batteries midday, you can effectively combat fatigue and stay alert throughout your day.

Enhancing Productivity

Next, let us delve into how short naps can positively impact productivity. Maintaining optimal productivity levels can be challenging in an era of constant hustle and bustle. However, several studies, including research published in The Guardian, have linked short naps to increased productivity (Davis, 2023).

This productivity swell can be attributed to the refreshing effect of naps on the mind and body. Short naps relieve fatigue, restore energy, and refresh the mind, enabling you to tackle tasks more efficiently. Consequently, you will likely produce higher quality work and achieve your targets quicker post-nap. So, the next time you feel your productivity waning, consider taking a short power nap instead of reaching for that cup of coffee.

Improving Attention Span

Finally, let us explore the power of naps in improving attention span. An overloaded mind can severely impact your ability to focus, leading to a dwindling attention span. A study found that taking a nap counteracts impulsive behavior and improves tolerance for frustration (Cheng et al., 2015).

In essence, a short nap acts like a system reboot, clearing unnecessary information and leaving the mind fresh to absorb new data. This rejuvenation enhances cognitive function and improves concentration, ultimately extending your attention span. Therefore, a well-timed short nap can be a significant game-changer in activities that require sustained attention.

In conclusion, short naps are a potent tool, enhancing alertness, boosting productivity, and improving attention span. Incorporating these brief bouts of rest into your routine allows you to maximize your potential and navigate your day with renewed energy and focus.

Techniques for Effective Power Napping and Optimal Nap Duration

Dive into the art of power napping with this guide to effective napping techniques and optimizing your nap duration for maximum benefits.

The Ideal Duration of a Power Nap

Once a dedicated night owl, Oscar found himself in a constant battle against fatigue. His job demanded sharp focus and quick decision-making, but his exhaustion increasingly shadowed his performance. Then, he stumbled upon an article about power napping and its benefits, particularly the significance of timing.

Power napping, Oscar learned, revolved around the clock. Napping too long could lead to grogginess, while too short might yield insufficient rejuvenation. The sweet spot? A mere 10 to 20 minutes. Intrigued and desperate for relief, Oscar incorporated this seemingly simple technique into his daily routine.

The initial attempt was rough. His mind seemed intent on running a marathon of thoughts rather than resting. But, with patience and consistency, Oscar began to master the art of the power nap. He set a strict limit of 15 minutes for his nap, armed with an alarm to rouse him from sleep.

Over time, Oscar noticed an impressive difference. No longer did he fight to keep his eyes open during afternoon meetings. He was alert, able to contribute fresh ideas and quick solutions. The previously insurmountable fog of fatigue began to lift. The power nap had quickly become his secret weapon.

Oscar's newfound alertness was not just psychological. According to research, power napping for 10 to 20 minutes allowed him to enter stage two of the sleep cycle, enhancing attention and concentration (Lawler, 2023). Going beyond 20 minutes could lead him into a deep sleep, making him wake up in a state of sleep inertia.

Oscar also found that the timing of the nap was critical. Mid-afternoon, when the body naturally experiences a dip in circadian rhythm, was ideal. He set a recurring calendar reminder for his power nap, holding that time sacred just as he would for an important meeting.

Throughout his journey, Oscar learned that everyone's sleep needs are unique, and the ideal duration could vary. However, the 10–20-minute power nap stood out as a potent tool for rapid rejuvenation.

The impact of power napping extended far beyond his professional life. His quick catnaps sparked a positive ripple effect, bringing vibrancy back into his personal life. Evenings no longer meant slumping on the couch, fighting sleep. He was present, engaged, and full of life.

Oscar's story illustrates the immense potential of power napping when done right. The optimal nap duration can act as a lever, pulling you up from the depths of fatigue and propelling you forward with renewed energy and focus. It is an accessible tool waiting to be wielded by anyone yearning for improved alertness and productivity in their day-to-day life.

Aided by the power of short naps, Oscar transformed his life, weaving productivity and well-being into a balanced tapestry. He became a living testament to the importance of quality rest, even if it was just for a few minutes a day.

Tips for Creating a Nap-Friendly Environment

Danielle, a hardworking entrepreneur, always sought ways to maximize her productivity. Despite her best efforts, she often felt drained and sluggish in the afternoon. Research led her to power napping, a strategic short rest to revitalize the mind. Keen to try it, Danielle created the perfect environment for her power naps.

Firstly, Danielle understood that finding a suitable space was crucial. She set her sights on creating a quiet area devoid of distractions. This meant converting a small corner of her office into her nap zone at work. She added a comfy couch, a cozy throw blanket, and even a fluffy eye mask to shield her from the ambient office lighting.

Danielle also recognized the importance of temperature control. Research suggested that a cooler room facilitated better sleep, so she adjusted her office thermostat to a slightly cooler temperature during her nap times. Danielle found that this slight adjustment enhanced her comfort and ability to fall asleep quickly.

Noise control was Danielle's next focus. She started using noise-canceling headphones to block out the ambient sounds in her workspace. On days when she found it particularly hard to wind down, she used a white noise app on her phone. The soothing, consistent sound acted like an auditory blanket, wrapping her in comfort and making her transition to sleep smoother.

However, setting up the perfect environment did not mean power napping was an instant success. In the initial stages, Danielle struggled. She consistently reminded herself to treat the nap as a brief pit stop, not a lengthy hiatus. It was a challenging shift in mindset, but gradually she began to appreciate the short, rejuvenating breaks.

Soon, Danielle found her rhythm. Her nap-friendly environment was working its charm. The quiet corner became a sanctuary where she could temporarily disconnect from her fast-paced routine. She found herself more energized and attentive post-nap, and she could even tackle complex tasks with newfound vigor.

As an entrepreneur, Danielle also saw potential beyond her personal benefit. She recognized that her employees, too, could benefit from power naps. Thus, she extended her initiative to the entire office, providing a dedicated quiet room for employees to use for power napping.

The introduction of the nap-friendly environment brought about a noticeable shift in office dynamics. Danielle noticed that her team appeared more energized and productive, especially in the post-lunch slump that usually drained their efficiency. The shared experience of power napping also created camaraderie among team members.

Through her journey, Danielle discovered that power napping was more than just closing her eyes for a few minutes. It involved creating the right environment—quiet, comfortable, and inviting—that supported her journey to quick, refreshing slumbers. She came to appreciate that small environmental tweaks could significantly increase her workday productivity and overall well-being.

Now a staunch advocate for power napping, Danielle often shares her experience with other entrepreneurs. She encourages them to look beyond traditional productivity techniques and consider the power of rest. Danielle's nap-friendly environment is a testament to the fact that power naps, when done right, can serve as a vital tool in one's productivity arsenal.

Did You Know?

It is fascinating that some individuals dream solely in black and white. Studies have linked this phenomenon to exposure to black-and-white television or film media. Those who grew up before color television was typical often report dreaming in black and white. This implies our dreaming minds may be influenced by the visual stimulation we receive when awake (feather&black, n.d.).

Are you still battling to fall asleep? Then try the method below.

Sleep Remedy One: Coffee Nap

Consider consuming a cup of coffee immediately before indulging in a brief 15- to 20-minute power nap. Given that the stimulating effects of caffeine typically start after around 20 minutes, you will awaken to the combined invigorating impacts of the rest and your coffee.

Sleep Remedy Two: Energizing Fruit Smoothie

Blend together a ripe banana, a handful of different berries, a tablespoon of nut butter, and a splash of almond milk. Enjoy as a refreshing and nourishing snack before a power nap. The ripe banana offers a natural source of tryptophan, which can help relax the body and promote sleepiness.

The assortment of berries, rich in antioxidants, supports brain health and may aid in reducing stress levels for better rest. Nut butter adds healthy fats and protein, providing sustained energy and helping to stabilize blood sugar levels during your power nap. Almond milk contributes magnesium, promoting muscle relaxation and potentially improving the quality of your short nap. While sipping that delicious smoothie close your eyes and imagine the beautiful waves crashing against the sandy coast, and picture palm tree branches swaying in the wind. Before you know it, you may find yourself in the middle of the best nap of your life!

The last chapter in our journey together will be about exploring actionable sleep solutions for different age categories. See you there.

Chapter 10:

Sleep Solutions for All Ages

Sleep is an investment in the energy you need to be effective tomorrow. –
Tom Roth

Discover practical, nurturing strategies to enhance your infant's sleep, fostering healthy sleep habits early on for optimal growth and well-being.

Sleep Solutions for Infants

Join us as we unpack proven strategies to improve your infant's sleep. Geared for children aged 0–12 months, these techniques foster healthy development and serene nights.

Sleeping Patterns and Needs of Infants

Understanding infant sleep patterns, typically erratic during the first few months, is essential for new parents. Newborns sleep about 16–17 hours a day, distributed unevenly over a 24-hour period. As infants grow, night sleep lengthens, and day sleep consolidates into naps. By six months, most infants sleep about 14 hours daily with two naps. Remember, each baby is unique. While adhering to general guidelines, be observant and responsive to your baby's individual needs. Recognizing these patterns and adapting strategies accordingly ensures a balanced sleep routine, fostering optimal health and development for your little one.

Creating a Safe and Soothing Sleeping Environment for the Tiny Humans

A safe, soothing sleep environment is crucial for your infant's restful slumber. Start by ensuring their crib meets safety standards, with a proper mattress and a fitted sheet. Keep it free from toys, pillows, or heavy duvets to decrease the risk of sudden infant death syndrome (SIDS). Use a room temperature between 68–72°F, avoiding overheating. Implement a calming bedtime routine—a warm bath, gentle massage, or a soft lullaby can work wonders. A white noise machine can emulate the womb's sounds, promoting comfort. By cultivating this serene environment, you encourage healthy sleep patterns for your tiny human, ensuring their well-being and development.

Healthy Sleep Routines for Infants

Establishing healthy sleep routines for your infant can shape their sleep habits for years to come. Initiate a consistent bedtime and wake-up time, even on weekends. Incorporate soothing activities like reading a story or humming a soft tune to signal it is time to sleep. During the daytime, engage your baby in stimulating play to differentiate between day and night. Feed them upon waking rather than at sleep times to disconnect sleep from feeding. Be patient, as routines take time to establish. Remember, your gentle, consistent efforts today pave the way for a lifetime of restful nights for your little one.

Infant Sleep Recipe

Try the solution below if your baby (and you) battle to have a peaceful night's rest.

Pour half a cup of finely milled oats into a sanitized baby tub or regular bathtub. Add warm water, carefully stirring to distribute the oats evenly. This comforting oatmeal bath, ideal before bedtime, can soothe your baby's senses, paving the way for tranquil sleep.

Did You Know?

An intriguing fact about infant sleep is that they do not differentiate between day and night sleep until about eight weeks old, which explains their varied sleep schedule (Better Health Channel, n.d.).

Sleep Solutions for Children

Next up, we explore practical strategies for children up to tweens, fostering healthy sleep habits that promote mental agility, physical health, and overall well-being.

The Importance of Consistent Sleep Schedules for Children

Consistent sleep schedules are vital for children aged one to twelve years. Regular bedtimes and wake times reinforce the body's natural circadian rhythm, promoting healthier, restful sleep. A consistent routine not only improves sleep quality but also benefits a child's overall development, enhancing their cognitive function, mood, and physical health. Bedtime rituals, like story reading or soft music, can signal sleep time, aiding in smoother transitions to sleep. Remember, consistency is key. Regularly adhering to sleep schedules, even during weekends, helps your child achieve optimal rest, setting them up for success in their waking hours.

Creating a Sleep-Friendly Environment for Children

Crafting a sleep-friendly environment propels your child toward restful nights. First, ensure their bedroom is dark, cool, and quiet—a setting conducive to sleep. Consider using blackout curtains and a white noise machine to block out disruptions. A comfortable, age-appropriate mattress and pillow add to their comfort. Keep the room clean and clutter-free, creating a calm space. Limit the bedroom to sleeping and relaxing activities, strengthening the association between bed and sleep. A nightlight or a comforting toy can address nighttime fears in older children. By fostering a sleep-friendly space, you empower your child for restorative sleep.

Relaxation Techniques and Bedtime Rituals for Children

Relaxation techniques and bedtime rituals can ease your child's transition to sleep. Start by creating a wind-down period, limiting stimulating activities to an hour before bed. Introduce calming practices like reading a favorite book together or gentle stretching exercises. Consider teaching older children simple mindfulness exercises, such as deep breathing or progressive muscle relaxation. These techniques can help them manage bedtime anxieties. A consistent bedtime ritual sends a powerful signal to your child's body that it is time to sleep. Each soothing step, from brushing teeth to saying goodnight, helps establish a sense of security and routine, promoting deeper, more restful sleep.

Sleep Recipe for Children

Use this awesome remedy for your pre-teenaged kids.

Combine one ripe banana, a cup of your chosen milk (dairy or plant-based), a spoonful of nut butter, a pinch of cinnamon, and a touch of honey in a blender. Process until silky smooth. This bedtime smoothie, with the soothing properties of cinnamon and natural sugars from the banana, is an inviting sleep inducer for your child. Serve it before their sleep time for a tranquil night.

The ripe banana provides tryptophan, an amino acid that supports the body in producing serotonin and melatonin, hormones that regulate sleep. The chosen milk offers calcium, which contributes to the body's sleep-wake cycle. Nut butter adds healthy fats and protein, promoting steady energy levels throughout the night. Cinnamon's calming properties may help reduce restlessness, and honey's natural sugars provide a gentle energy source that aids in relaxation. Together, these ingredients create a delicious and sleep-enhancing treat for children. Always ensure the recipe is suitable for your child's dietary preferences and any potential allergies.

Did You Know?

Fascinatingly, by the age of two, most children have spent more time asleep than awake in their lifetime, and overall, a child will spend 40% of their childhood sleeping (Cooper, 2020).

Sleep Solutions for Teenagers

Unearth effective sleep strategies for teenagers aged 13 to 19 to foster restful nights and vibrant days for this critical developmental stage.

Sleep Challenges Specific to Teenagers

This life stage, aged 13–19, often faces unique sleep challenges. The onset of puberty triggers a shift in their circadian rhythms, causing a natural preference for late bedtimes and morning sleep-ins. This misaligns with early school start times, leading to sleep deprivation. Additionally, societal pressures, academic stress, and an increase in electronic device usage can further disrupt sleep. Understanding these challenges is the first step in addressing teenage sleep issues. Encouraging good sleep hygiene, maintaining a regular sleep schedule, and fostering a sleep-friendly environment can help teens navigate these challenges and achieve the sleep they need for optimal health and growth.

Limiting Tech Use and Its Impact on Sleep in Teens

Limiting tech use among teenagers is crucial for their sleep health. The blue light released from electronic devices can suppress melatonin. This can lead to delayed sleep onset and reduced sleep quality. Encourage teens to disconnect from electronics at least an hour before bedtime. Consider designating tech-free zones, like the bedroom, to minimize distractions. Also, promote other calming, nonscreen activities such as reading or journaling. By managing tech use, we can help our teenagers harness the power of restorative sleep, thereby supporting their overall well-being and development.

Healthy Sleep Habits and Stress Management for Teens

Promoting healthy sleep habits and stress management techniques can significantly improve a teenager's sleep quality. Encourage regular sleep schedules, even on weekends, to align their biological clocks. A clean, dark, and quiet sleep environment can foster restful sleep. Consider teaching teens relaxation techniques like yoga, mindfulness, or deep breathing exercises to manage stress effectively. Regular physical activity can also aid in stress relief and promote better sleep. These practices and open discussions about their stressors can empower teenagers to manage their stress levels, leading to healthier sleep patterns and improved overall well-being.

Sleep Recipes for Teenagers

This remedy is specially crafted for sleeplessness in teens.

Blend together a ripe banana, a handful of spinach, a few slices of kiwi, a tablespoon of chia seeds, and a splash of coconut water. Enjoy it as a calming and nutritious treat before winding down for sleep.

The ripe banana offers tryptophan, which can help regulate sleep and mood in teenagers. Spinach provides magnesium, supporting relaxation and muscle function, while also contributing to overall health. Kiwi contains serotonin-boosting nutrients and antioxidants that may aid in reducing stress, promoting a peaceful mindset before bedtime. Chia seeds are rich in omega-3 fatty acids, contributing to brain health and potentially enhancing sleep quality. Coconut water provides hydration and electrolytes, ensuring teenagers stay refreshed and relaxed as they prepare for sleep.

Bonus Remedy: Teenage Bedtime Smoothie

Blend together 1 cup of Greek yogurt, 1 ripe banana, a handful of mixed berries, a tablespoon of chia seeds, and a drizzle of honey. Enjoy this nutrient-packed smoothie as a wholesome and delicious evening treat.

The Greek yogurt offers protein and calcium, which can help regulate sleep patterns and support bone health during the crucial teenage years. The ripe banana provides natural sugars and tryptophan, contributing to relaxation and potential sleep enhancement. Mixed berries are rich in antioxidants, assisting in reducing oxidative stress and promoting overall well-being, which is important for growing teenagers. Chia seeds are a great source of omega-3 fatty acids and fiber, aiding in satiety and providing a slow-release energy source throughout the night. The touch of honey not only adds sweetness but may also have mild sedative properties, promoting relaxation and sleep readiness.

Did You Know?

Interestingly, during adolescence, a teenager's circadian rhythm undergoes a "phase delay," causing them to naturally feel alert later at night and wake up later in the morning, often conflicting with early school start times (Moawad, 2016).

Sleep Solutions for Adults

Discover actionable sleep strategies for adults aged 20 and beyond, promoting restorative sleep essential for maintaining physical health and cognitive function.

Sleep Hygiene and Bedtime Routines for Grownups

Good sleep hygiene and consistent bedtime routines are invaluable for adults seeking quality sleep. Sticking to sleep and wake times, even on weekends, help regulate your body's internal clock. Create a sleep-friendly environment—quiet, dark, and cool, with comfortable bedding. Engage in relaxing activities before sleep, such as listening to a bedtime story for adults, not eating dinner too late, or dimming the lights as soon as it gets dark. Limit exposure to screens before bed to limit the onslaught of blue light on melatonin. Adults can improve sleep, cognitive function, mood, and overall health by prioritizing these habits.

Managing Stress and Anxiety for Improved Adult Sleep

Effective stress and anxiety management play a pivotal role in improving adult sleep. Establishing a regular exercise routine aids in stress relief and promotes restful sleep. Consider practicing mindfulness techniques, like blindfolded movement or pinwheel breathing exercises, to help quiet the mind and alleviate anxiety. Maintain a positive sleep environment, free from work or other stress-inducing elements. Encourage open conversations about mental health and consider professional help if anxiety becomes overwhelming. Managing stress and anxiety not only helps in enhancing sleep quality but also contributes significantly to your overall mental and physical well-being.

Creating a Comfortable Environment for Optimal Rest

Crafting a comfortable environment is integral to achieving optimal rest. For ideal sleep conditions, your bedroom should be cool, around 60–67°F. Invest in high-quality mattresses, pillows, and bedding that suit your comfort preferences. Consider using blackout curtains, an eye mask to block light, earmuffs, or a colored noise machine to mute disruptive sounds. To foster a stress-free space, keep your room tidy and free from work-related materials. By nurturing this sleep-friendly sanctuary, you encourage your body and mind to relax and unwind, facilitating deep, restorative sleep.

Sleep Recipes for Adults

Below is a soothing sleeping remedy for adult insomniacs.

Sauté ground turkey in a pan until it's well-cooked and exhibits a golden-brown hue. Flavor with salt, pepper, and a selection of your favorite herbs or spices for added taste. Lay crisp lettuce leaves on a platter and spoon the flavorful turkey onto each leaf. This light yet protein-dense dinner offers an excellent prebedtime meal. Tryptophan, found abundantly in turkey, aids in producing serotonin, a sleep-enhancing hormone, thereby encouraging a good night's rest.

Bonus Remedy: Warm Lavender Epsom Salt Bath

Dissolve 1 cup of Epsom salt and a few drops of lavender essential oil in a warm bath. Soak for 20 minutes before bed. Epsom salt provides magnesium, while lavender's aroma promotes relaxation.

Did You Know?

Interestingly, while it's a common belief that adults need less sleep as they age, the National Sleep Foundation maintains that adults (26–64 years) should aim for seven to nine hours of sleep, similar to younger adults (18–25 years; Pacheco, 2020).

Sleep Solutions for Seniors

Explore effective sleep strategies for seniors aged 65 and above, essential for maintaining health, cognitive function, and overall quality of life.

Understanding Age-Related Changes in Sleep Patterns for Older Adults

As we age, changes in sleep patterns become evident. Seniors often experience earlier bedtimes and wake times due to shifts in their internal biological clocks. They may also wake up frequently during the night and have overall lighter sleep. Understanding these age-related sleep changes is crucial in addressing sleep issues among seniors. Tailored sleep strategies can mitigate these changes, such as keeping a consistent sleep schedule and establishing a sleep-friendly environment. Promoting healthy sleep in seniors contributes to their physical health, cognitive function, and overall well-being.

Addressing Common Sleep Disorders in Seniors

Seniors commonly face sleep disorders like insomnia, sleep apnea, RLS, and circadian rhythm sleep disorders. Acknowledging and addressing these disorders is vital for their sleep health. Regular exercise can help manage symptoms of insomnia and RLS. For sleep apnea, maintaining a healthy weight and avoiding alcohol can be beneficial. When circadian rhythms are disrupted, light therapy can be an effective solution. A healthcare professional should always guide treatment strategies. Timely intervention and proper management of these sleep disorders can enhance a senior's sleep quality and significantly improve their quality of life.

Gentle Relaxation Techniques and Exercise for Improved Senior Sleep

Gentle relaxation techniques and regular exercise can significantly enhance sleep quality in seniors. Incorporating low-impact activities like walking, swimming, or listening to night sounds in daily routines can facilitate better sleep. Practices like listening to delta-frequency binaural beats and steam inhalation can also help induce relaxation and reduce anxiety before bedtime. Additionally, listening to a sleep podcast can promote better sleep by easing stress and calming the mind. Encouraging these healthy lifestyle habits contributes to improved sleep in seniors and supports their overall physical and mental well-being, enhancing their quality of life.

Sleep Recipes for Seniors

Find below the perfect sleeping remedy for older adults.

Warm a mugful of your preferred milk—be it cow's or plant-based—on the stove, ensuring it does not reach boiling point. Mix in a dash of nutmeg, blending thoroughly. Sip this comforting beverage before sleep. Nutmeg, known for its soothing qualities, can assist seniors in achieving relaxation and restful sleep.

Bonus Remedy: Senior Bedtime Ritual

Engage in a calming bedtime routine that includes gentle stretching, reading a soothing book, and a cup of chamomile tea. These activities can help seniors unwind and prepare for a restful night's sleep.

The gentle stretching exercises relax the body, improve flexibility, and promote blood circulation, contributing to a more comfortable sleep experience for seniors. Reading a soothing book can calm the mind and divert it from any worries, aiding in reducing anxiety and facilitating sleep.

Chamomile tea, known for its mild sedative properties, can help alleviate restlessness and promote relaxation, which is particularly beneficial for seniors who may experience sleep disturbances.

Did You Know?

Interestingly, seniors spend more time in the lighter stages of sleep than in deep sleep. This change in sleep architecture could be a reason why older adults may experience frequent awakenings throughout the night (Li et al., 2018).

Recipes Disclaimer: Always engage with a healthcare provider for individualized guidance and to confirm the appropriateness of proposed remedies or recipes, particularly if you are managing existing health conditions or are on prescribed medications.

Conclusion: Embracing Your Restful Sleepscape

It is a common experience that a problem difficult at night is resolved in the morning after the committee of sleep has worked on it. –John Steinbeck

As we come to the end of this journey through the realm of sleep, I hope you have found a deeper understanding of its fundamental role in our lives. Sleep, often underestimated, is the key to unlocking a healthier, more fulfilled, and ultimately more productive version of ourselves. Through these pages, we have explored the mystery of sleep, delving into its fascinating mechanisms and intricate processes that significantly influence both our physical and mental well-being.

Each chapter has been meticulously crafted to arm you with practical, accessible strategies to optimize the quality of your rest. These are not mere theories but solid, proven, science-backed principles that stand to revolutionize your relationship with sleep. The importance of understanding sleep cannot be overstated. It is the lifeline that supports the entirety of our existence—our health, cognitive function, emotional balance, creative spirit, and even our mood and outlook on life.

We have explored the importance of an optimal sleep environment, shedding light on the often neglected aspects of our sleeping quarters. Every detail plays an indispensable role, from lighting and noise control to the quality of our bedding and the temperature. You now have an army of tools at your disposal to turn your bedroom into a sanctuary conducive to the deepest, most restful sleep.

Further, we have journeyed through the maze that is stress management, a vital aspect of improving our sleep quality. Stress and sleep share a bidirectional relationship, affecting the other in multiple ways. By practicing mindfulness, relaxation techniques, and other stress-reducing activities, we can break this cycle and foster an environment of peace and calm.

Our journey did not stop there. We also delved deep into the importance of sleep hygiene, exploring habits that promote quality sleep. From managing our exposure to screens before bed to establishing a consistent sleep schedule, we have detailed the crucial practices that help regulate our internal clock and promote a healthier sleep cycle.

Continuing our journey, we must pause to consider the power of quality sleep. It is not just about the number of hours we clock in but the quality of those hours. Deep, restorative sleep promises rejuvenated energy, enhanced productivity, and a sense of serenity. As we have learned, sleep is not a passive process but an active and essential function responsible for crucial tasks such as memory consolidation, cell repair, and detoxification.

Each chapter has unraveled these complex processes, illuminating the importance of each stage of the sleep cycle. The remarkable world of REM and non-REM sleep and the integral functions they perform were examined. With this newfound understanding, you can begin to appreciate how each night's sleep serves as a vital journey for your mind and body.

Diving into the sea of sleep disorders, this book has also cast light upon conditions that can rob us of quality sleep. Insomnia, sleep apnea, RLS, and more were explored not just to raise awareness but to equip you with knowledge. Acknowledging such conditions is the first step toward seeking professional help, and this book serves as your guide in identifying symptoms and understanding treatments.

This understanding extends beyond yourself. It provides a perspective to empathize with loved ones who may be struggling, enabling you to offer support and guide them toward the help they need. Sleep disorders are not just personal battles but collective issues that impact relationships, productivity, and societal health.

As we dove deeper, we unearthed the undeniable relationship between sleep and other aspects of our lives—our dietary habits, physical activity, and mental health. The profound impact of nutrition on rest was dissected, and you are now armed with many recipes promoting sleep. Integrating these sleep-enhancing foods into your daily routine enables you to craft a diet that supports restful sleep.

Moreover, we highlighted the role of physical activity in regulating our sleep-wake cycle. Exercise is not only for weight management or cardiovascular health; it is a potent tool for sleep optimization. By participating in regular physical activity in your daily routine, you take a significant stride towards quality sleep.

And let us not forget the essential role of mindfulness and mental health in sleep quality. From art therapy and sleep hypnosis audio therapy to cognitive behavioral therapy, we have discussed the myriad ways to harness the power of our minds to enhance our sleep. By managing stress and nurturing mental well-being, you can eliminate many sleep disturbances and move toward restorative sleep.

In essence, the journey toward restful sleep is a holistic one. It encompasses every aspect of our routines, environment, habits, and mental health. The journey does not end here. As you turn this last page, a new chapter in your life begins. It is a chapter where you take charge of your sleep, decide to prioritize this vital aspect of health, step away from sleepless nights and step into a world of refreshing, rejuvenating slumber.

You have now been introduced to a myriad of recipes and remedies, curated with care, to supplement your sleep improvement journey. These wholesome, sleep-friendly nutritional ideas serve to align your dietary habits with your sleep health. Restful sleep is as much about what we do during the day as at night.

And so, dear reader, you stand equipped, ready to usher in a new era of restful, rejuvenating sleep into your life.

This book, however, is not just a guide—it is a catalyst for change. It is an invitation to step into the world of mindful sleeping, where every night is a nurturing retreat. But the onus to enact this transformation lies with you. As you turn the last page, remember that the most profound journeys begin with a single step.

Start tonight. Make that one small change. Dim the lights an hour before bed. Turn off your electronic devices. Or perhaps, try that chamomile tea recipe you read about. Step by step, night by night, allow the insights from this book to guide you.

You are on the precipice of unlocking the secrets to restorative rest. Don't merely survive on minimal, fitful sleep—thrive on quality rest. Embrace the science of sleep and embark on this transformative journey. Your path to a healthier, more rejuvenating sleep life begins now.

Now, insomniac, the baton is passed on to you. You hold the key to unlock a world of restorative rest. The wisdom gleaned from these pages is only as potent as your commitment to apply it.

As you close this book, open your mind and heart to change. Start small. Choose one strategy, one recipe, one change, and begin there. Ingrain it into your routine until it becomes a part of you. Then move on to the next. With each small victory, you will find yourself inching closer to your goal—restorative sleep, waking up each morning with renewed energy, and living your life not in a fog of fatigue but with clear, focused vitality.

So, embark on this exciting journey. Be patient with yourself, for change is a process, not an event. Remember, the secret to transforming your sleep lies not in the grand, sweeping changes but in the small, consistent steps.

The path to restful sleep is paved with conscious choices, mindful habits, and a deep understanding of sleep's intrinsic value. Embrace this journey with open arms. As you traverse this path, know that each step you take is a move toward a healthier, happier, and more fulfilling life.

In your hands lies the power to transform your nights and, with it, your days. As you conclude this reading, I invite you to step into the world of mindful sleep. The journey to restorative sleep starts now. Embrace the night, welcome the dawn, and celebrate the gift of restful sleep. Your better life begins tonight.

And always remember, every good day starts with a good night. Sleep well.

Celebrities Who Credit Sleep to Their Success

Jeff Bezos—Amazon Founder

Known worldwide as the powerhouse behind Amazon, Jeff Bezos is a living testament to the transformative power of ambition, innovation, and a good night's sleep. The journey of Bezos, from a Wall Street computer science whiz to the helm of a trillion-dollar company, is a riveting saga. However, it is worth noting that amid all the business strategy and technological wizardry, the magnate places high importance on restful sleep.

Born in the year 1964 in Albuquerque, New Mexico, Bezos showed an early flair for mechanics and technological inventiveness. He excelled academically, eventually reaching Princeton University, earning an electrical engineering and computer science degree. Following a stint on Wall Street, Bezos established Amazon.com, an online bookseller, in 1994. His small startup rapidly blossomed into an e-commerce juggernaut, transforming how we shop, read, and engage with technology.

Bezos credits much of his success to prioritizing a whole night's sleep, usually clocking in around eight hours a night. He said, "Eight hours of sleep makes a big difference for me, and I try hard to make that a priority" (Medium, 2016).

He firmly believes that getting sufficient rest improves the quality of his decisions. For him, making a few high-quality decisions is more critical than making numerous good ones, and sleep plays a pivotal role.

Being an industry leader demands mental sharpness, creative thinking, and the ability to make crucial decisions, all of which Bezos links directly to his sleep quality. He has often shared his philosophy that maintaining a healthy work-life harmony, which includes adequate rest, contributes to increased productivity and creativity.

For Bezos, sleep is not just a biological necessity but a strategic tool for success. He rejects the stereotype of the constantly hustling entrepreneur who survives on minimal sleep. Instead, he emphasizes the need for leaders to take care of their physical well-being to stay effective. He realizes that his sleep pattern significantly affects his mood, vitality, and business acumen.

In a world that often celebrates grueling work schedules, Bezos sets a different tone. He starts his days free of early morning meetings, allowing for a calm and unhurried start after a whole night's sleep. He also encourages the same philosophy within his team at Amazon, promoting a work culture that respects the need for rest and recovery.

His commitment to adequate rest also influences his broader leadership strategies. He prioritizes a "work hard, have fun, make history" ethos in his company, promoting a balanced lifestyle for his employees. This approach has paid off as Amazon continues to lead the way in technological innovations and customer service.

Jeff Bezos' success story is extraordinary in many ways. However, the Amazon CEO's insistence on the benefits of a good night's sleep adds an essential element to his narrative. By underscoring the impact of rest on creativity, decision-making, and overall productivity, Bezos illustrates that success is not just about hard work and intelligent strategies; it's also about ensuring that we prioritize our physical well-being and understand the science of sleep.

Jennifer Lopez—Dancer, Singer, and Actress

Jennifer Lopez, affectionately known as J.Lo, is a global sensation. With a career spanning music, film, fashion, and television, her success is a testament to hard work, creativity, talent, and the power of a good night's sleep. Her journey, from a humble upbringing in the Bronx to global stardom, inspires many.

Born in 1969, Lopez showed early inklings of her love for the performing arts. Her Puerto Rican mother and father encouraged her and her siblings to pursue their artistic passions. J.Lo took to dancing, singing, and acting like a natural, quickly proving herself a triple threat.

She initially gained recognition as a dancer on *In Living Color*, but her breakout role as Selena Quintanilla in the 1997 biopic *Selena* marked her ascent to stardom. A string of successful movies followed, but Lopez wasn't content with just acting. She ventured into music, releasing her debut album *On the 6* in 1999. The album's lead single, "If You Had My Love," skyrocketed to the top of the Billboard charts, setting the stage for J.Lo's illustrious music career.

Lopez soon became a global superstar with her sizzling dance moves, powerful voice, and charismatic acting. But what is her secret to maintaining such high energy levels? A full night's sleep.

Lopez has long espoused the benefits of quality sleep, usually aiming for nine to ten hours each night. She often credits her age-defying looks and energy levels to her dedication to a healthy lifestyle, of which sleep is crucial.

She says, "The number one tip is to always get enough sleep. I can't stress this enough. Ideally, I would love to get nine or ten hours of sleep, but either way, I always make sure I get at least eight" (GRAZIA, 2021).

Her commitment to sleep is part of a broader philosophy of self-care and wellness. For J.Lo, fitness, a healthy diet, and quality sleep go hand in hand, forming the bedrock of her productivity and performance. She ensures her evenings are dedicated to winding down, creating an atmosphere conducive to a peaceful night's sleep.

Lopez also believes that sleep is crucial to her creative process. The mental clarity, focus, and energy derived from a restful sleep enhance her performances, whether on stage, in front of a camera, or while penning a new song.

J.Lo defies the norm in an industry that often glorifies nonstop hustle, underscoring the importance of restorative sleep. Her philosophy is simple: Taking care of yourself is the first step to success.

Today, Jennifer Lopez's name is synonymous with success, but she still remembers sleep's essential role in her journey. Her dedication to balancing hard work and adequate rest is a powerful lesson for those aspiring to shine in their respective fields.

Bill Gates—Microsoft Founder

Bill Gates, one of the most influential figures of our era, has shaped the course of technology and philanthropy with a unique blend of vision, innovation, and an unyielding dedication to a full night's sleep. His journey from a curious teenager to a tech giant and philanthropist is one of purpose, resilience, and well-rested cognition.

Born in 1955 in Seattle, Washington, Gates developed an early interest in computing while studying at Lakeside School. He wrote his first software program at the tender age of 13. He cofounded Microsoft with his childhood friend Paul Allen in 1975, beginning an incredible journey to revolutionize personal computing.

From Microsoft's first operating system, MS-DOS, to the iconic Windows and the suite of Office products, Gates led the company with a clear vision and deep understanding of the burgeoning digital age. But as Microsoft grew, so did Gates' commitment to his sleep routine.

Gates firmly believes in the power of a good night's sleep and has often highlighted its role in his success. He aims for at least seven hours of sleep each night, considering it not a luxury but a necessity for maintaining his productivity, creativity, and decision-making skills.

He says, "I like to get seven hours of sleep a night because that's what I need to stay sharp and creative and upbeat" (Umoh, 2017). Gates' respect for sleep aligns with his meticulous approach to his work and life, which revolves around constant learning, analysis, and reflection.

The emphasis on sleep is evident in his daily routines. Despite his packed schedule, Gates ensures he has a quiet, uninterrupted period before bedtime, often spent reading. This habit satiates his insatiable curiosity and helps him wind down, creating the right conditions for a rejuvenating sleep.

Gates recognizes the role of sleep in fostering cognitive abilities. He understands that the brain uses rest to consolidate learning, an essential aspect of his work where innovation is the lifeblood. It is not just about keeping his energy levels high; it is about optimizing his intellectual power.

In 2006, Gates transitioned from Microsoft to the Bill and Melinda Gates Foundation, channeling his energy into addressing global challenges. His zeal for problem-solving and strategizing, backed by restful sleep, has enabled him to tackle complex issues, from education reform to health initiatives.

Even when addressing global issues or discussing future plans, Gates does not dismiss the importance of sleep. His message to aspiring leaders and entrepreneurs is clear: Respecting your sleep is respecting your success.

Today, as one of the world's wealthiest and most influential individuals, Gates continues to inspire millions. His success is not just a testament to his visionary leadership and relentless drive but also to his balanced lifestyle, with sleep playing a pivotal role.

LeBron James—Professional Basketball Player

LeBron James, a name synonymous with power, prowess, and an unyielding drive for excellence, dominates not just on the basketball court but also the world of sleep. As a four-time NBA champion, two-time Olympic gold medalist, and 17-time All-Star, LeBron's commitment to a solid night's sleep has played a pivotal role in his towering success.

Welcomed to the world on December 30, 1984, in Akron, Ohio, LeBron's journey from a struggling neighborhood to the zenith of the basketball world reflects a tale of determination, grit, and extraordinary talent. He spent his high school years shattering records, commanding national attention, and earning the title of "the best high school basketball player in America" (Langridge, 2020).

The Cleveland Cavaliers welcomed LeBron into the NBA in 2003, and his career took flight. His unmistakable talent, paired with a relentless work ethic, propelled him to become one of the greatest basketball players of all time. However, behind his monumental success lies a lesser-known secret - his unwavering dedication to a restful night's sleep.

LeBron James ardently believes in the power of sleep, famously admitting to averaging 12 hours of sleep per day—a significant contrast to the average American's 6.8 hours (Lee, 2017). His sleep regime may seem lavish, but LeBron understands its importance in achieving peak performance. While we sleep, our bodies recover, restoring and rejuvenating muscles that endure grueling training sessions. For an athlete of LeBron's caliber, this recovery is non-negotiable.

He credits his longevity in the physically demanding world of professional basketball to prioritizing sleep. LeBron's commitment is so firm that he invested in optimizing his sleep environment. He employs top-notch sleep technologies and therapies, including a custom-designed bed and a sound-proof, temperature-controlled room. Moreover, despite his chaotic travel schedule, he practices sleep hygiene techniques like maintaining a consistent bedtime.

LeBron's cognizance of sleep's impact on performance extends beyond physical recovery. He recognizes sleep influences cognitive functions such as decision-making and reaction times - elements integral to his game. His dominating on-court presence, instantaneous decision-making, and lightning-quick responses are partly a testament to his healthy sleep habits.

Moreover, LeBron's focus on sleep has garnered attention in the sports science world. His performance sheds light on the correlation between optimal sleep and athletic performance, influencing a paradigm shift where rest is recognized as an essential component of training regimens.

LeBron's sleep habits also have a spillover effect on his off-court activities. Being a tireless advocate for social justice, an active businessman, and a dedicated family man requires immense energy. Adequate sleep ensures that he is always at the top of his game, regardless of whether he is making a play or closing a business deal.

From humble beginnings to present-day dominance, LeBron James continues to illustrate that his commitment to peak performance transcends the basketball court. It permeates every facet of his life, with sleep at the heart of his endeavors. His story underlines a powerful message: Success is not merely about talent or training but also hinges on restful, restorative sleep.

Tom Brady—Football Star

Tom Brady, one of the best footballers of all time, has a secret weapon that is not so secret: a full night's sleep. Brady, who is often held in high regard for his discipline, perseverance, and leadership, also credits sleep as a significant contributor to his long-standing career and remarkable achievements.

Born in 1977 in California, Brady's passion for football was palpable early on. After participating in college football at Michigan, he was drafted by the New England Patriots in 2000. Initially underestimated as the 199th pick, Brady quickly rose through the ranks, shattering expectations and carving out an illustrious career.

Brady's leadership led the Patriots to win six Super Bowls, making him a household name and an emblem of success in the National Football League (NFL). Despite changing his team to the Tampa Bay Buccaneers in 2020, his winning streak remained unbroken, clinching yet another Super Bowl victory in 2021.

Behind Brady's impressive on-field performance lies a rigorous commitment to wellness, in which sleep plays a pivotal role. Brady strongly believes in the power of a good night's sleep and ensures he gets at least eight to nine hours per night. He views sleep as a time for his body to recover from the strains of a highly physical sport and to rejuvenate for optimal performance.

"Proper sleep has helped me get to where I am today as an athlete," Brady explains, "and it is something that I continue to rely on every day" (Wallace, 2017).

As part of his sleep regimen, Brady adheres to a strict bedtime routine, retiring before 9 p.m. and waking up at 5:30 a.m. This discipline extends to his presleep rituals too. He ensures a technology-free, calming environment and incorporates various recovery tools like bioceramic sleepwear to enhance sleep quality.

Brady's emphasis on the importance of sleep extends beyond personal practice. He often shares his sleepcentric approach with his teammates, encouraging them to prioritize restful sleep to elevate their performance. This underscores his commitment to sleep and his leadership quality, advocating for a team that's rested and ready to conquer the field.

From the early days of his career to his consistent successes as an accomplished football player, Brady's commitment to quality sleep stands out as a cornerstone of his success. It illustrates that the foundation of athletic excellence is not solely training and skill but also includes holistic wellness practices like restful sleep.

Today, Brady's name continues to echo in the stadiums, and his story continues to inspire. He has transformed his discipline, perseverance, and sleep-centric wellness approach into a lifestyle brand, TB12, advocating a holistic approach to athletic performance.

Brady's success story is a testament to his talent, determination, and priority for sleep. It is a clear message to aspiring athletes that a path to greatness involves rigorous training, a competitive spirit, and the often-underestimated power of sleep.

References

17 calming activities before bedtime. (2018, April 2). Harmony. https://harmonylearning.com.au/17-calming-activities-before-bedtime/

6 steps to better sleep. (2020, April 17). MAYO CLINIC. https://www.mayoclinic.org/healthy-lifestyle/adult-health/in-depth/sleep/art-20048379

10 curious facts about sleep. (n.d.). Feather&Black. https://www.featherandblack.com/online-features/inspiration/10-curious-facts-about-sleep

22 facts about sleep that will surprise you. (2021, March 1). Cleveland Clinic. https://health.clevelandclinic.org/22-facts-about-sleep-that-will-surprise-you/

Abbasi, B., Kimiagar, M., Sadeghniiat, K., Shirazi, M. M., Hedayati, M., & Rashidkhani, B. (2012). *The effect of magnesium supplementation on primary insomnia in elderly: A double-blind placebo-controlled clinical trial.* Journal of Research in Medical Sciences: The Official Journal of Isfahan University of Medical Sciences, 17(12), 1161–1169. https://www.ncbi.nlm.nih.gov/pmc/articles/PMC3703169/#:~:text=Conclusion%3A

Ackerman, C. (2017, January 18). *22 mindfulness exercises, techniques & activities for adults (+ pdfs).* PositivePsychology.com. https://positivepsychology.com/mindfulness-exercises-techniques-activities/

AlShareef, S. M. (2022). *The impact of bedtime technology use on sleep quality and excessive daytime sleepiness in adults.* Sleep Science, 15, 318–327. https://doi.org/10.5935/1984-0063.20200128

Anxiety disorders. (2022, April). National Institute of Mental Health. https://www.nimh.nih.gov/health/topics/anxiety-disorders

Bardo, N. (2021, July 11). *Perfect sleep: How to create the best nighttime routine.* It's ALL YOU Boo. https://itsallyouboo.com/create-best-night-time-routine-for-adults/

Bauer, B. (2017). *Pros and cons of melatonin.* MAYO CLINIC. https://www.mayoclinic.org/healthy-lifestyle/adult-health/expert-answers/melatonin-side-effects/faq-20057874

Bechtel, W. (2015). *Circadian rhythms and mood disorders: Are the phenomena and mechanisms causally related?* Frontiers in Psychiatry, 6. https://doi.org/10.3389/fpsyt.2015.00118

BedBreeZzz Media. (n.d.). *"Go to bed you'll feel better tomorrow" is the human version of "Did you try turning it off and on again?"* Pinterest. https://za.pinterest.com/pin/755971487440614917/

Behavioral intervention improves sleep for hospitalized pregnant women. (2017, December 18). American Academy of SLEEP MEDICINE. https://aasm.org/sleep-hygiene-improves-sleep-pregnant-women/

Blue light has a dark side. (2020, August 13). Harvard Health Publishing. https://www.health.harvard.edu/staying-healthy/blue-light-has-a-dark-side

Boyle, N., Lawton, C., & Dye, L. (2017). *The effects of magnesium supplementation on subjective anxiety and stress—A systematic review.* Nutrients, 9(5), 429. https://doi.org/10.3390/nu9050429

Brain basics: Understanding sleep. (2022, September 26). National Institute of Neurological Disorders and Stroke. https://www.ninds.nih.gov/health-information/public-education/brain-basics/brain-basics-understanding-sleep

Breus, Michael. J. (2017). *Your guide to better sleep.* SLEEP DOCTOR. https://thesleepdoctor.com/

Cain, Á. (2017, January 19). *5 successful people who always get a full night of sleep.* INSIDER. https://www.businessinsider.com/successful-people-who-sleep-2017-1#jeff-bezos-2

Carolyn Dean quote: "Magnesium oil has the ability to increase the body's production of DHEA, a hormone that has beneficial effects on memory..." (n.d.). Quotefancy. https://quotefancy.com/quote/2238681/Carolyn-Dean-Magnesium-oil-has-the-ability-to-increase-the-body-s-production-of-DHEA-a

CDC - Sleep home page - Sleep and sleep disorders. (2019). Centers for Disease Control and Prevention. https://www.cdc.gov/sleep/index.html

Chang, A.-M., Aeschbach, D., Duffy, J. F., & Czeisler, C. A. (2014). *Evening use of light-emitting eReaders negatively affects sleep, circadian timing, and next-morning alertness.* Proceedings of the National Academy of Sciences, 112(4), 1232–1237. https://doi.org/10.1073/pnas.1418490112

Chaput, J.-P., McHill, A. W., Cox, R. C., Broussard, J. L., Dutil, C., da Costa, B. G. G., Sampasa-Kanyinga, H., & Wright, K. P. (2022). *The role of insufficient sleep and circadian misalignment in obesity.* Nature Reviews Endocrinology. https://doi.org/10.1038/s41574-022-00747-7

Cheng, P., Kemp, K., Caccamo, L., Roberts, J., & Deldin, P. (2015, June 29). *Feeling impulsive or frustrated? Take a nap.* ScienceDaily. https://www.sciencedaily.com/releases/2015/06/150629111059.htm

Circadian rhythms. (2020). National Institute of General Medical Sciences. https://www.nigms.nih.gov/education/fact-sheets/Pages/circadian-rhythms.aspx

Colten, H. R., Altevogt, B. M., & Research, I. of M. (US) C. on S. M. and. (2006). *Sleep physiology.* In www.ncbi.nlm.nih.gov. National Academies Press (US). https://www.ncbi.nlm.nih.gov/books/NBK19956/#:~:text=NREM%20sleep%20constitutes%20about%2075

Cooper, J. (2020, July 20). *Why is sleep important for our health?* Lewisham Children and Family Centres. https://www.lewishamcfc.org.uk/why-is-sleep-important-for-our-health/

Costello, R. B., Lentino, C. V., Boyd, C. C., O'Connell, M. L., Crawford, C. C., Sprengel, M. L., & Deuster, P. A. (2014). *The effectiveness of melatonin for promoting healthy sleep: A rapid evidence assessment of the literature.* Nutrition Journal, 13(1). https://doi.org/10.1186/1475-2891-13-106

Cousins, J. N., Wong, K. F., Raghunath, B. L., Look, C., & Chee, M. W. L. (2018). *The long-term memory benefits of a daytime nap compared with cramming.* Sleep, 42(1). https://doi.org/10.1093/sleep/zsy207

Davis, N. (2023, June 23). *Calls to make nap part of working day after latest study on brain benefits.* The Guardian. https://www.theguardian.com/lifeandstyle/2023/jun/23/calls-nap-sleep-work-study-research-benefits

Dement, W. C., & Vaughan, C. C. (2000). *The promise of sleep: A pioneer in sleep medicine explores the vital connection between health, happiness, and a good night's sleep.* Dell Trade Paperback.

Fritscher, L. (2020, May 15). *How the collective unconscious is tied to dreams, beliefs, and phobias.* Verywellmind. https://www.verywellmind.com/what-is-the-collective-unconscious-2671571

Global insomnia statistics in 2022. (n.d.). Helsestart. https://www.helsestart.no/news/global-insomnia-statistics

Goel, N., Basner, M., Rao, H., & Dinges, D. F. (2013). *Circadian rhythms, sleep deprivation, and human performance.* Progress in Molecular Biology and Translational Science, 119, 155–190. https://doi.org/10.1016/b978-0-12-396971-2.00007-5

Green, E. (2012, June 4). *A bedtime routine for adults: 10 relaxing activities for sleep.* NO SLEEPLESS NIGHTS. https://www.nosleeplessnights.com/bedtime-routine-for-adults/

Hackett, R. A., Dal, Z., & Steptoe, A. (2020). *The relationship between sleep problems and cortisol in people with type 2 diabetes.* Psychoneuroendocrinology, 117, 104688. https://doi.org/10.1016/j.psyneuen.2020.104688

Hale, L. (2018). *Youth screen media habits and sleep.* Child and Adolescent Psychiatric Clinics of North America, 27(2), 229–245. https://doi.org/10.1016/j.chc.2017.11.014

Hall, A. (2014, April 28). *14 highly successful people who prioritize a good night's sleep.* HUFFPOST. https://www.huffpost.com/entry/successful-people-who-sle_n_5201290

Happy. (2022, August 15). *What is the activation-synthesis theory of dreaming?* Psychcrumbs. https://psychcrumbs.com/what-is-the-activation-synthesis-model-of-dreaming/#:~:text=The%20activation%2Dsynthesis%20theory%20is

Helmer, J. (2022, September 22). *Reducing the effects of blue light.* WebMD. https://www.webmd.com/eye-health/blue-light-reduce-effects#:~:text=Adding%20a%20screen%20filter%20to

How Jennifer Lopez's body at 51 is stronger than her body at 30. (2021, January 12). GRAZIA. https://graziamagazine.com/us/articles/jennifer-lopez-exercise-diet-regime/#:~:text=%E2%80%9CThe%20number%20one%20tip%20is

Jeff Bezos: Why getting 8 hours of sleep is good for Amazon shareholders. (2017, April 27). Medium. https://medium.com/thrive-global/jeff-bezos-sleep-amazon-19c617c59daa#:~:text=Jeff%20Bezos%3A%20Eight%20hours%20of

Jewett, B. E., & Thapa, B. (2020). *Physiology, NMDA Receptor.* National Center for Biotechnology Information; StatPearls Publishing. https://www.ncbi.nlm.nih.gov/books/NBK519495/

Juma, N. (2021, March 26). *Sleep quotes honoring powerful rest and relaxation.* EVERYDAYPOWER. https://everydaypower.com/sleep-quotes/

K, V., & A, R. (2009). *The threat simulation theory in light of recent empirical evidence: A review.* The American Journal of Psychology. https://pubmed.ncbi.nlm.nih.gov/19353929/

Kaur, H., Spurling, B. C., & Bollu, P. C. (2020). *Chronic insomnia.* PubMed; StatPearls Publishing. https://www.ncbi.nlm.nih.gov/books/NBK526136/

Kim, E.-J., & Dimsdale, J. E. (2007). *The effect of psychosocial stress on sleep: A review of polysomnographic evidence.* Behavioral Sleep Medicine, 5(4), 256–278. https://doi.org/10.1080/15402000701557383

Langridge, M. (2022, May 30). LeBron James net worth, height, wife, news & more. DMARGE. https://www.dmarge.com/who-is-lebron-james

Lashbrooke, B. (2019, August 20). *When it comes to sleep, are you an Ellen DeGeneres, Mariah Carey, or Margaret Thatcher?* Forbes. https://www.forbes.com/sites/barnabylashbrooke/2019/08/20/when-it-comes-to-sleep-are-you-an-ellen-degeneres-or-a-marissa-mayer/?sh=87c7ed82299b

Lawler, M. (2023, June 20). *Do power naps actually work?* Everyday Health. https://www.everydayhealth.com/sleep/power-naps-the-benefits-how-long-they-should-be-and-when-they-work-best/

Lazzerini Ospri, L., Prusky, G., & Hattar, S. (2017). *Mood, the circadian system, and melanopsin retinal ganglion cells.* Annual Review of Neuroscience, 40(1), 539–556. https://doi.org/10.1146/annurev-neuro-072116-031324

Lee, B. Y. (2017, June 9). This is how many hours of sleep Lebron James gets a day. Forbes. https://www.forbes.com/sites/brucelee/2017/06/09/this-is-how-many-hours-of-sleep-lebron-james-gets-a-day/?sh=245e64179b2c

Li, J., Vitiello, M. V., & Gooneratne, N. S. (2018). *Sleep in normal aging.* Sleep Medicine Clinics, 13(1), 1–11. https://doi.org/10.1016/j.jsmc.2017.09.001

Li, Q., Keohane, L. M., Thomas, K., Lee, Y., & Trivedi, A. N. (2017). *Association of cost-sharing with use of home health services among medicare advantage enrollees.* JAMA Internal Medicine, 177(7), 1012. https://doi.org/10.1001/jamainternmed.2017.1058

Lindberg, S. (2019, November 22). *Autogenic training: What it is and how to do it.* Healthline. https://www.healthline.com/health/mental-health/autogenic-training

Lovato, N., & Lack, L. (2010). *The effects of napping on cognitive functioning.* Progress in Brain Research, 185, 155–166. https://doi.org/10.1016/B978-0-444-53702-7.00009-9

Magnesium. (2022, June 2). Office of Dietary Supplements. https://ods.od.nih.gov/factsheets/Magnesium-HealthProfessional/#:~:text=Magnesium%20is%20a%20cofactor%20in

Marturana Winderl, A. (2021, July 22). *11 soothing nighttime habits for restful sleep and a productive next morning.* SELF. https://www.self.com/story/pre-sleep-habits

Melatonin: What you need to know. (2022, July). National Center for Complementary and Integrative Health. https://www.nccih.nih.gov/health/melatonin-what-you-need-to-know

Meyer, N. (2014, January 13). *The NASA studies on napping.* PRICECONOMICS. https://priceonomics.com/the-nasa-studies-on-napping/#:~:text=The%20NASA%20team%20concluded%20that

Moawad, H. (2016, November 7). *Teenage circadian rhythm.* NeurologyLive. https://www.neurologylive.com/view/teenage-circadian-rhythm

Murphy, A. (2020, April 1). *11 relaxing activities before bed to fall asleep fast.* Declutter the Mind. https://declutterthemind.com/blog/relaxing-activities-before-bed/

Newsom, R. (2020, November 4). *Blue light: What it is and how it affects sleep.* SLEEP FOUNDATION. https://www.sleepfoundation.org/bedroom-environment/blue-light#:~:text=Inversely%2C%20exposure%20to%20blue%20light

Olson, E. J. (2021, May 15). *How many hours of sleep do you need?* MAYO CLINIC. https://www.mayoclinic.org/healthy-lifestyle/adult-health/expert-answers/how-many-hours-of-sleep-are-enough/faq-20057898

Pacheco, D. (2020, November 13). *Memory & sleep: How deprivation affects the brain.* SLEEP FOUNDATION. https://www.sleepfoundation.org/how-sleep-works/memory-and-sleep

Pacheco, D. (2023). *Bedroom environment: What elements are important?* SLEEP FOUNDATION. https://www.sleepfoundation.org/bedroom-environment

Patel, A. K., Reddy, V., & Araujo, J. F. (2022, September 7). *Physiology, sleep stages.* PubMed; StatPearls Publishing. https://www.ncbi.nlm.nih.gov/books/NBK526132/#:~:text=Sleep%20occurs%20in%20five%20stages

Pickering, G., Mazur, A., Trousselard, M., Bienkowski, P., Yaltsewa, N., Amessou, M., Noah, L., & Pouteau, E. (2020). *Magnesium status and stress: The vicious circle concept revisited.* Nutrients, 12(12), 3672. https://doi.org/10.3390/nu12123672

Potter, J. D., Robertson, S. P., & Johnson, J. D. (1981). *Magnesium and the regulation of muscle contraction.* Federation Proceedings, 40(12), 2653–2656. https://pubmed.ncbi.nlm.nih.gov/7286246/

Quotes about insomnia: The best of. (2021, January 7). BetterSleep. https://www.bettersleep.com/blog/insomnia-quotes/

Relaxation techniques: Try these steps to reduce stress. (2022). MAYO CLINIC. https://www.mayoclinic.org/healthy-lifestyle/stress-management/in-depth/relaxation-technique/art-20045368

Scipioni, J. (2021, February 6). *A 9 p.m. bedtime and special pajamas: Inside Tom Brady's sleep routine.* CNBC. https://www.cnbc.com/2021/02/06/-inside-tom-bradys-sleep-routine.html

Sleep. (n.d.). Healthychildren.org. https://www.healthychildren.org/English/healthy-living/sleep/Pages/default.aspx

Sleep deprivation and deficiency - What are sleep deprivation and deficiency? (2022, March 24). National Heart, Lung, and Blood Institute. https://www.nhlbi.nih.gov/health/sleep-deprivation

Sleep disorders. (n.d.). MedlinePlus. https://medlineplus.gov/sleepdisorders.html#:~:text=There%20are%20more%20than%2080

Spirtzler, F. (2018, August 22). *10 magnesium-rich foods that are super healthy.* Healthline; Healthline Media. https://www.healthline.com/nutrition/10-foods-high-in-magnesium

Summer, J. (2020, October 9). *Napping: Health benefits & tips for your best nap.* SLEEP FOUNDATION. https://www.sleepfoundation.org/sleep-hygiene/napping

Suni, E. (2020a). *What is circadian rhythm?* (A. Dimitriu, Ed.). SLEEP FOUNDATION. https://www.sleepfoundation.org/circadian-rhythm

Suni, E. (2020b, August 14). *What is sleep hygiene?* (N. Vyas, Ed.). SLEEP FOUNDATION. https://www.sleepfoundation.org/sleep-hygiene

The interpretation of dreams. (n.d.). FREUD MUSEUM LONDON. https://www.freud.org.uk/education/resources/the-interpretation-of-dreams/#:~:text=Freud%20called%20dream%20interpretation%20the

Tryptophan. (2013). MedlinePlus. https://medlineplus.gov/ency/article/002332.htm

Typical sleep behaviour (1) – newborns 0 to 3 months. (n.d.). Better Health Channel. https://www.betterhealth.vic.gov.au/health/healthyliving/typical-sleep-behaviour-nb-0-3-months

Umoh, R. (2017, August 2). *Billionaires Jeff Bezos and Bill Gates say they work best after a full night's rest.* CNBC. https://www.cnbc.com/2017/08/02/jeff-bezos-and-bill-gates-say-they-work-best-after-sleeping.html

Understanding the stress response. (2020, July 6). Harvard Health Publishing. https://www.health.harvard.edu/staying-healthy/understanding-the-stress-response

Wahl, S., Engelhardt, M., Schaupp, P., Lappe, C., & Ivanov, I. V. (2019). *The inner clock—Blue light sets the human rhythm.* Journal of Biophotonics, 12(12). https://doi.org/10.1002/jbio.201900102

Walker, M. P. (2017). *Why we sleep: Unlocking the power of sleep and dreams.* Scribner, An Imprint Of Simon & Schuster, Inc.

Walker, W. H., Walton, J. C., DeVries, A. C., & Nelson, R. J. (2020). *Circadian rhythm disruption and mental health.* Translational Psychiatry, 10(1). https://doi.org/10.1038/s41398-020-0694-0

Wallace, B. (2017, January 11). *Tackling tech: Tom Brady, smart clothes, and the pursuit of peak performance.* PATRIOTS. https://www.patriots.com/news/tackling-tech-tom-brady-smart-clothes-and-the-pursuit-of-peak-performance-286981#:~:text=%22I%20firmly%20believe%20that%20sleep

Wamsley, E. J. (2014). *Dreaming and offline memory consolidation. Current Neurology and Neuroscience Reports, 14(3).* https://doi.org/10.1007/s11910-013-0433-5

West, M. (2022, April 21). *Guided imagery: Techniques, benefits, and more.* MEDICALNEWSTODAY. https://www.medicalnewstoday.com/articles/guided-imagery

YourQuote: India's largest writing app. (n.d.). YOURQUOTE. https://www.yourquote.in/

Printed in Great Britain
by Amazon

31405068R00086